SUPER-POWERED
IMMUNITY

SUPER-POWERED
IMMUNITY

Natural Remedies for 21st-Century Viruses and Superbugs

Michelle Schoffro Cook, Ph.D., DNM

Healing Arts Press
Rochester, Vermont

Healing Arts Press
One Park Street
Rochester, Vermont 05767
www.HealingArtsPress.com

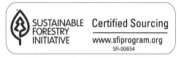

Text stock is SFI certified

Healing Arts Press is a division of Inner Traditions International

Note to the reader: This book is intended as an informational guide. The remedies, approaches, and techniques described herein are meant to supplement, and not to be a substitute for, professional medical care or treatment. They should not be used to treat a serious ailment without prior consultation with a qualified health care professional.

Cataloging-in-Publication Data for this title is available from the Library of Congress

ISBN 978-1-64411-602-9 (print)
ISBN 978-1-64411-603-6 (ebook)

Printed and bound in the United States by Lake Book Manufacturing, LLC
The text stock is SFI certified. The Sustainable Forestry Initiative® program promotes sustainable forest management.

10 9 8 7 6 5 4 3 2 1

Text design and layout by Kenleigh Manseau
This book was typeset in Garamond Premier Pro with Elza used as display typefaces

To send correspondence to the author of this book, mail a first-class letter to the author c/o Inner Traditions • Bear & Company, One Park Street, Rochester, VT 05767, and we will forward the communication, or contact the author directly at **DrMichelleCook.com**.

Contents

Acknowledgments

To my husband, for your love, support, and for always picking up the slack while I write books

To my family, for your love and support: Bobbi-Jo Meyer, Michael and Deborah Schoffro

To Jon Graham, for your belief in this project and me as an author

To all the people at Inner Traditions who contributed their skills and expertise to this book

To the many wonderful and highly-skilled herbalists who have inspired my quest for herbal knowledge over the years, including Dr. Cobi Slater, Robert Rogers, Beverley Gray, and Rosemary Gladstar

Introduction

Discover a New World of Immune-Enhancing Remedies

Viruses and superbugs have become a part of day-to-day living, but that doesn't mean you have to live in fear of those nasty microbes. Your immune system, when armed with nature's best weapons, can be a formidable rival against a wide range of viruses and bacteria. However, not just any remedy will do. *Super-Powered Immunity: Natural Remedies for 21st-Century Viruses and Superbugs* reveals the most valuable natural remedies and their powerful healing abilities.

In this groundbreaking book, you'll discover the best herbs, essential oils, mushrooms, probiotics, and other powerful options to protect you from a host of viruses and superbugs—even those resistant to antibiotics and other drugs! When I tell people that there are natural remedies that work even when the drug options do not, I am inevitably asked: "Why hasn't my doctor told me about them?" or "Why hasn't my doctor prescribed them?" Many people wrongly believe that if their doctor hasn't prescribed these natural remedies, they must not actually be helpful. But that couldn't be further from the truth. These natural medicines offer the solutions that most medical doctors are unaware of because, sadly, few medical doctors have received training in this field.

Instead, most doctors rely heavily on their pharmaceutical-based training and drug options. These laboratory-derived pharmaceutical drugs have their shortcomings, not the least of which is that they are chemically simplistic in their structures, making it easy for superbugs to figure them out and become resistant to them—a serious and growing problem we're currently facing. Few people, medical doctors included, realize that the most powerful natural medicines are actually much more chemically complex than those synthetically produced ones created by pharmaceutical companies.

In contrast, many of the natural medicines I have curated and feature in *Super-Powered Immunity* are far more chemically complex than pharmaceutical options, making them very difficult for superbugs to outsmart! And, of course, the natural choices have far fewer, if any, side effects.

There are many other books on immunity in the marketplace, most of which claim that ordinary foods, nutrients, and lifestyle changes can boost immunity. While this is true and certainly advisable, in reality, most of these options are only minimally effective when facing a severe viral or bacterial infection. The most powerful natural remedies that really *can* supercharge the immune system are frequently omitted from most books, and rarely ever make it into blogs on the topic. When it comes to fighting a superbug, these omissions can spell the difference between health and long-term illness, or worse.

You'll find that the dietary and lifestyle recommendations, as well as the super-powered immune boosters that I include in this book, must meet rigorous research and clinical standards. Unfortunately, I have found no other natural healing books that include critical information on essential oils, herbs, mushrooms, and probiotics—the "big guns" when it comes to immunity.

I've spent nearly three decades tracking down the most effective natural weapons against viruses and bacteria. What led me to do this? What led me to undertake this search? In fact, it was my own survival.

When I discovered that, like millions of others worldwide, I had severe allergic reactions to many common drugs, I committed to seeking natural options to restore my health. In the process, I gained unique expertise in the field of natural healing and immunity, not just from my research, but also in using my body as a living laboratory.

Even with remedies that are in common use, I often found that people didn't use them in the best ways to optimize their efficacy, which sometimes meant contracting infections they might not have otherwise gotten, difficulty overcoming infections that lingered longer or were more troublesome than they needed to be, or just a low-functioning and vulnerable immune system.

Most people take remedies in insufficient doses, without adequate frequency, or in an incorrect form, which usually results in either minimal effectiveness or no noticeable results at all. It is critical to identify the most powerful remedies (including the correct species when it comes to plants) and the most effective form of the remedy (such as infusion, tincture, oil extract, or another form). It is also critical to ensure that it is used in a correct dosage amount and with the ideal frequency and duration to yield the best healing results.

Yet, most people merely dabble without consideration as to whether they're using the wrong plant species, in a minimally effective format, in insufficient doses, often enough to yield results. Over the years, I've heard many people claim that they've "tried everything," but upon examination of their efforts, it turns out that they lacked the knowledge to implement the use of particular remedies or used ineffective options. Alternatively, they may have opted for a remedy that was a powerful antibacterial remedy but hadn't shown much activity against viruses— the issue they were facing. So, it was no surprise that they didn't get the results they had hoped for.

In *Super-Powered Immunity,* I'll arm you with the knowledge of research-supported remedies and how to use them to get results against bacterial, fungal, and viral threats, even superbugs that have outsmarted antibiotics and other drugs.

In chapter 1, you'll learn how the immune system works, and why it is more important than ever to boost it as we face growing threats from viruses, superbugs, and pandemics. This is particularly true because viruses and superbugs mutate, coming back in different forms, so keeping your immune system strong is the best way to ensure you're ready for anything.

In chapter 2, you'll discover which foods are the best ones to fortify your immune system and keep infections at bay. From old standbys like garlic and ginger to lesser-known immune boosters like turmeric, you'll create the foundation for great immune health. You'll also learn about key nutrients and how to take them for the best results. Some of these remedies include: glutathione, N-acetyl cysteine, vitamin C, vitamin D, quercetin, and zinc, to name a few. You'll learn why the government-recommended daily intakes are a joke as well as the ideal amount to supplement with for powerful immunity against infections.

In chapter 3, you'll find the best researched, natural, antiviral and antibacterial herbs and essential oils, like chamomile, garlic, ginger, star anise, and thyme; the best forms of each to take; and how to use them to reap the greatest health benefits. In this chapter, you may be surprised to learn that certain essential oils (not all!) are the real powerhouses to overcome viral and bacterial threats. You'll find out why essential oils, which are between fifty and seventy times stronger than their herbal counterparts, are some of the most overlooked yet most powerful immune-boosting remedies when used correctly. (Hint: most people don't use them to maximize their immune-boosting benefits!) You'll learn how to safely benefit from essential oils like cinnamon, cloves, melaleuca (tea tree), oregano, star anise, thyme, and many others.

In chapter 4, I'll share why the idea of killing *all* bacteria in the body has led to superbugs that have outsmarted our best drugs. This is known as "antibiotic resistance." I'll share the exciting new research that shows that restoring beneficial bacteria—*probiotics*—can help strengthen the body's immune system, fight harmful bacteria, and go to battle against viruses. You'll learn about the best strains of beneficial bacteria that help ensure their proliferation in the body.

In chapter 5, medical and clinical research continues to reveal the power of mushrooms like reishi, chaga, lion's mane, turkey tail, and shiitake to supercharge your immune system. You'll also learn how to get more of these immune-boosting superstars into your diet and supplements.

In chapter 6, you'll find out about the common dietary and lifestyle habits that knock out your immune system, often for hours at a time, leaving you vulnerable to viral or bacterial infections, and how to incorporate simple but powerful strategies to supercharge your immune system for life. You'll learn how to create a lifestyle that will raise your odds of super-powered immunity for life.

Armed with *Super-Powered Immunity,* you can benefit from these discoveries of these foods, herbs, essential oils, nutrients, mushrooms, and other immune-boosting remedies with my recommendations for ensuring their maximum effectiveness. It is my hope that the healing wisdom found in these pages will serve you for years to come. As humanity enters the ever-changing landscape of viral challenges and antibiotic-resistant bacteria, this book will be just as valuable in the future as it is today. Unlike many drugs whose potency against super-bugs is questionable or waning, the natural remedies throughout this book have been in use in many cases for thousands of years and are still as effective as when our ancient ancestors used them.

Welcome to a new world of vital immune-enhancing possibilities and potent opposition against harmful microbes.

1
Uncover Your Powerful Immune Response

The Importance of Super Immunity

A friend shared that she read a newspaper story in which a medical doctor claimed to have discovered the key to overcoming the Covid-19 pandemic. Excited to learn more, I asked her to share the doctor's discovery. She said that the medical doctor quoted throughout the news story seemed to think that the immune system was the key to overcoming the recent viral challenges our world faced.

I waited for her to share some novel piece of information, anticipating that somewhere in the conversation she would finally get to the heart of the matter—some exciting new discovery. When it became clear to me that the article author, and the medical doctor cited in the story, were enthralled with their "discovery" that the immune system could overcome viral threats, something that they considered a new discovery, I was quickly disappointed.

After all, our immune system is as old as humanity itself. The fact that we are alive on the planet is a testament to the immune systems of our ancestors working at peak function to overcome the viral, bacterial, fungal, or parasitic threats their bodies faced. And, they did so long before the advent of pharmaceutical drugs that even the oldest of which have only been around for a hundred or so years. Most drugs have only been around for much less than that.

Your immune system, when equipped with the tools it needs to do its job, can overcome even the worst threats. But, it needs support to ensure optimal functioning. You'll discover why you should build your immune system's strength, as well as the best ways to do so, in the following chapters.

But first, let's explore the immune system and how it works so you'll be better able to improve its functioning to fight off even the worst threat. Most of us have heard of the immune system and realize that it is important to our health, but few people actually know what it is, which is obvious by my friend's report of the medical doctor and news reporter who seemed to think they had made a significant discovery against viral illnesses.

WHAT EXACTLY IS MY IMMUNE SYSTEM?

Your immune system is your body's defense against infection and disease. It evaluates substances floating around your body, assessing whether they are supposed to be there or not, whether they are naturally part of your body or a foreign intruder that poses a risk to your health.

While there are many components of the immune system, there are five main ones, which include:

Bone Marrow: Marrow is a soft, spongy tissue that is primarily located inside the larger bones of the body, including the arms, legs, vertebrae, and pelvis in your body. While we think of our bones as fairly static, they hold an important part of our immune system. The red marrow produces red and white blood cells. The yellow marrow helps in the production of white blood cells. These blood cells help to fight against invaders in the body.

Lymphatic System: A vast network of lymph nodes and vessels that carry lymphatic fluid, nutrients, and waste products between your bodily tissues and bloodstream. The lymph nodes filter the fluid that passes between them, capturing viruses, bacteria, and other foreign invaders, which are then destroyed by cells known as lymphocytes.

Spleen: The spleen is a fist-sized organ on the left side of your abdomen. It filters the blood by removing old or damaged cells, while also destroying bacteria and other foreign invaders that may otherwise compromise your health.

Tonsils and Thymus: The tonsils are the two small oval masses of tissue at the back of your throat, and the thymus is a gland in your upper chest behind your ribs. They are responsible for producing antibodies, which are combatants against foreign invaders in your body.

White Blood Cells: Made in the bone marrow, these cells attack and destroy organisms, such as bacteria, viruses, or other microbes, that could threaten your health.[1]

Immune system cells, which are needed to do battle against germs, are made in various parts of your body, including the adenoids, bone marrow, lymph nodes, lymphatic vessels, Peyer's patches, the spleen, the thymus, and tonsils.[2] While some of these elements were explored above, some of these may be unfamiliar.

Adenoids: Your adenoids are two glands found at the back of your nasal passages.

Lymph nodes: Tiny organs shaped like beans, the lymph nodes are located throughout your body and are connected via an intricate lymphatic network.

Lymphatic vessels: Your lymphatic vessels carry immune cells known as lymphocytes to the bloodstream and throughout your body.

Peyer's patches: Peyer's patches are tissue that is found in your small intestines.

The Common Cold

20 Signs You Have an Upper Respiratory Infection and What to Do About It

No one likes having a cold. You know why: the pressure in the head, the sinus congestion that frequently feels unending, and then there's the coughing . . . the seemingly unceasing coughing. Unless the symptoms hit like a ton of bricks though, it's not always obvious whether your symptoms are due to allergies or sinusitis, or if it's actually an upper respiratory infection (URI), also known as the common cold.

There are many signs or symptoms of the common cold or an upper respiratory infection. It is not necessary to have all of them for a cold to be present, but the following symptoms are the most common:

Bad Breath

Body Aches

Burning Eyes

Coughing

Excessive Mucus

Eye Irritation

Eye Redness

Facial Pain

Facial Pressure

Fever (may or may not be present, more common with children, tends to reflect flu rather than a cold)

Headaches

Itchy Eyes

Loss of Sense of Smell

Nasal Congestion

Runny Nose

Scratchy Throat

Sneezing

Sore Throat

Swelling and/or Discomfort of the Nasal Passageways

Why You Should Stop Demanding Antibiotic Prescriptions for Your Cold

While many doctors still hand out prescriptions for antibiotics like they are candy, they do not work against the common cold, which is usually viral in nature. Antibiotics, like the name suggests (anti-bacteria), only work against bacterial infections, not those with a viral origin.

So, before you visit your doctor demanding a prescription for antibiotics for your cold you may want to consider that:

1. It will be a waste of your time;
2. It will be a waste of your money;
3. It won't end your misery; and
4. It will contribute to the growing number of superbugs that have become antibiotic-resistant largely due to the over-prescription of antibiotics. These superbugs are leading to infections that can cause serious health problems and even death so it is best not to contribute to the serious problem we are now facing.

According to the Lucille Packard Children's Hospital at Stanford, there are over two hundred viruses that can cause upper respiratory infections. According to the same organization, it is estimated that in any year-long period, Americans collectively suffer around one billion colds. A group of viruses called rhinoviruses are largely to blame for colds. The average adult has between two and four colds per year while children get six to eight colds annually, or more if they attend daycare.[3]

What Happens When You Catch a Cold

Once the virus enters your body either from droplets in the air or direct contact with someone who is infected, your immune system immediately goes to work, attacking it. The immune system's response results in an increase in mucus production causing a runny nose, swelling of the nose and nasal passageways causing congestion, irritation in the nose that causes sneezing, and an increased amount of mucus that drips down the throat and causes coughing. Symptoms usually begin within one to three days after contact with the virus.

Quick Ways to Ease Your Suffering

You'll find lots of remedies and strategies throughout this book to help you fight off a cold, or to prevent you from getting them in the first place. But, to help you get started, here are a few things you can do to ease your suffering:

Drink lots of fluids.

Get plenty of bed rest to allow your immune system to function optimally.

Take extra vitamin C (at least 500 mg, three times daily).

Use elderberry syrup to help with sore throats. Follow package directions.

Take oregano essential oil to help boost your immune system. Follow directions for the product you select.

Avoid dairy products since they add to the mucus in your body.

While we may come in contact with colds, that doesn't mean we have to excessively suffer. By adding a few natural remedies and ensuring adequate fluid and rest we can greatly reduce the amount or duration of suffering.

HOW CAN YOUR IMMUNE SYSTEM PROTECT YOU?

Now let's explore the workings of this critical system and discover why it is more important than ever to boost immunity as we face growing threats from viruses, superbugs, and pandemics.

Without a highly effective immune system, your body would have no way to fight off the harmful things that you come into contact with. Your immune system:

Fights disease-causing germs, also known as pathogens, which include: bacteria, fungi, and viruses;

Removes pathogens from your body;

Recognizes and neutralizes harmful substances from the environment; and

Fights disease-causing changes in the body, which includes cancer cells.[4]

The immune system is activated when it doesn't recognize something that is not your own cells or tissues, such as the proteins on the surfaces of bacteria, fungi, and viruses. These proteins are called antigens. When these antigens attach to the immune system cells, they trigger a series of processes that activate the immune system.

After the first contact with a disease-causing germ for the first time, the body's immune system stores information about the germ and how to fight it, enabling it to work faster and more effectively should it come into contact with this germ again in the future.[5] It's like your body has its own infectious disease-fighting repository of information so it can better handle infections the next time it comes across them.

Not only does this mechanism help your body ward off diseases it has already come into contact with, but it can help your body deal with pathogens as they mutate. As viruses and other germs mutate, which means that they come back in different forms, they pose new challenges to your immune system, but having information stored about the germs and how to fight them improves your immune system's ability to fight the mutated version in most cases. This is called "innate immunity."

Innate vs. Acquired Immunity

The various components of the immune system can be classified into two systems: the innate immune system and the acquired immune system. Your innate immune system is the inherent immunity you were born with. You were born with an immune system that can attack foreign invaders to help your body overcome them. It has been actively trying to keep you healthy from the day you were born. Whenever you come into contact with a foreign invader, whether it is a bacteria, fungus, or virus, your immune system springs into action to engulf the invader. Known as phagocytes, these front-line immune system cells actively work to kill off these harmful microbes.

The acquired immune system, with the help of the innate immune system, produce cells known as antibodies to protect your body from a specific invader. These antibodies are created in your body from cells known as B-lymphocytes after it has been exposed to a specific invader. For example, if your body came in contact with the SARS-CoV2 virus that caused Covid-19, your body's B-lymphocytes would work to create antibodies to help you overcome the viral threat. If you've ever heard someone say that they have antibodies to a particular illness, they are referring to these immune cells that are created by the immune system in response to coming into contact with a specific threat.

Antibodies can take several days to develop, but as soon as your immune system recognizes the invader, it immediately begins to attack it. Once it has the recognition of the particular invader, these antibodies can assist your body, should you ever come in contact with this particular pathogen again.

The innate immune system offers a general defense against harmful germs and substances, which is why it is also called the non-specific immune system. Don't mistake its generalized functioning with ineffectiveness because it is a highly powerful front-line system that fights off disease quickly and effectively in most cases, particularly when it is given all of the tools it needs to do so (we'll discuss more about these tools throughout this book). The innate immune system primarily fights using immune cells such as natural killer cells and phagocytes ("eating cells"). The innate immune system largely fights substances and germs that enter the body through the skin or digestive system.[6]

The "adaptive" or "acquired" immune system changes throughout your life as you come into contact with different bacterial, fungal, or viral threats, and as your body responds by making antibodies to overcome them. It's basically the storehouse of information on how to battle and win against whatever disease-causing germs you may have come into contact with.

The adaptive immune system makes antibodies, which it uses to fight specific germs that the body has previously been in contact with. Because part of the immune system is constantly learning, adapting, and evolving, the body can fight bacteria, fungi, or viruses that change over time, or "mutate."

WHEN THE IMMUNE SYSTEM ATTACKS HEALTHY TISSUE

While the immune system is a highly efficient system that keeps you alive and has ensured the survival of our ancestors for thousands of years, sometimes the body mistakes the proteins on the surface of its own cells for foreign cells and attacks them, which causes something known as an autoimmune response. There are many theories as to why this happens, including toxic build up in the cells or chemical food or drug ingredients that may disrupt the body's natural capacity to differentiate healthy from harmful cells or tissues, among others. Whole books could be written on the topic of autoimmune diseases, and indeed have been, so I won't be delving deeply into the topic here but you will find some information about remedies throughout *Super-Powered Immunity* that have been found effective at regulating the immune system.

THE GROWING THREAT OF SUPERBUGS

We keep hearing about "superbugs" but what exactly are they? Superbugs are strains of bacteria, fungi, parasites, and viruses that are resistant to most of the antibiotics (in the case of bacteria) or other medications that are commonly used to treat the infections caused by these microbes. They can cause a wide range of illnesses depending on the microbe, including: pneumonia or other respiratory infections like MRSA, skin infections, urinary tract infections (UTIs),[7] gonorrhea, or blood infections known as sepsis. Some of the resistant bacteria that can cause these infections include *Staphylococcus aureus* (*S. aureus*), *Klebsiella pneumoniae* (*K. pneumoniae*), *Escherichia coli* (*E. coli*), and *Clostridium difficile* (*C. diff.*), to name a few.

We are obsessed with germs. And, having just faced a pandemic, it is understandable that so many among us have made handwashing and sanitizing their favorite pastimes. While these measures certainly have their place and have helped many prevent the spread of harmful viruses, the sad reality is that our overuse of many antibacterial soaps, handwipes, cleaning products, and other antimicrobial items has actually helped to encourage the development of superbugs by exerting an evolutionary pressure against the infectious microbes that they must overcome for their survival. While their survival may be good news for infectious microbes, it tends to be bad news for humans as fewer of our drug-based medicines work against these heightened microbes that seemingly have a super capacity to survive.

Resistance, or drug resistance, or antimicrobial resistance, occurs over time. And, while it can happen naturally, it can be hastened or exacerbated by a wide variety of things that we do, without realizing that these habits or behaviors can be worsening drug resistance. While resistance can happen with any bacteria, fungi, or viruses, we have already seen the dangers of it linked to antibiotic resistance and the highly infectious bacteria that can result as we hear about increasing incidents of MRSA infections and other superbugs killing people in hospitals or other settings.

There are many ways that we may have unknowingly exacerbated antibiotic resistance, including: the overuse or overprescribing of antibiotics, misuse or mis-prescribing of antibiotics for non-bacterial infections, overuse of antibacterial consumer products, and flushing medications down the toilet where they will escape into waterways, to name a few.

We may not like to admit that we may have unknowingly played a role in the development of the superbugs that now challenge us, but we have. And, not just in the form of household cleaning products, hand soaps, and even air "disinfectants." Arguably, our overreliance and misuse of antibiotic drugs as well as our heavy-handed use of these drugs for veterinary purposes have been some of the main reasons for the rise of antibiotic resistance and the drugs' near extinction as the treatment of many disease-causing bacterial infections.

OUR WAR ON BACTERIA

We first began to understand bacteria in the 1800s thanks to Louis Pasteur who explored the possibility of germs in his germ theory of disease.[8] However, this concept of unseen creatures probably seemed ridiculous to physicians and the scientific community of the time. But after Pasteur, a chemist and physicist, lost three children to typhoid fever, he began exploring microbes, including bacteria and viruses. Typhoid fever is a disease caused by *Salmonella typhi* bacteria and is spread via contaminated water, other beverages, and food.[9] Without Pasteur's contribution to health and medicine, modern hygienic practices might never have evolved and surgeons would still be performing surgeries without washing their hands in advance.

Once the understanding of bacteria caught on, some scientists began studying the use of certain microbes to kill harmful bacteria. By 1928, Sir Alexander Fleming, a Scottish bacteriologist, pharmacologist, and botanist was studying influenza and he observed that mold had accidentally developed on his culture dishes in which he was growing staphylococci bacteria. He noticed that the mold had a bacteria-free circle around itself suggesting that it held some type of antibacterial properties and was killing the bacteria in its vicinity.

Further experimentation revealed that, indeed, mold could be used as a way to kill harmful bacteria, which led to the discovery of penicillin, an antibiotic drug that uses certain strains of mold to kill bacterial illnesses. Later, he was honored with a Nobel Prize for his discovery of penicillin.[10]

Another scientist, Robert Koch, is known as the father of modern bacteriology for his discoveries of the bacteria involved in tuberculosis, cholera, and anthrax.[11] He coined the term "antibiosis," which simply means "against life."

The explorations of how mold can kill bacteria led to antibiotics, which, for many years, have been our primary weapon against bacterial infections and the diseases linked to them.

OVERVIEW OF BACTERIA AND THEIR PRIMARY EFFECTS

Bacteria Type	Primary Effects
Acinetobacter baumanni	A. baumanni is an opportunistic microbe that often impacts people who are immunocompromised, particularly as skin or respiratory infections, and is frequently drug resistant.[12]
Escherichia coli	This frequently drug-resistant bacterium (commonly known as E. coli) is responsible for cramps, diarrhea, and vomiting linked to food poisoning and is frequently to blame (along with various species of Enterococcus bacteria) for UTIs.[13]
Helicobacter pylori	H. pylori is often implicated in ulcers and gastrointestinal health issues.
Mycobacteria	There are many species of bacteria collectively known as mycobacteria, some of which have been linked to conditions like leprosy and tuberculosis.[14]

OVERVIEW OF BACTERIA AND THEIR PRIMARY EFFECTS (*continued*)

Bacteria Type	Primary Effects
Pseudomonas aeruginosa	*P. aeruginosa* can cause infections in the eyes, blood, or respiratory system, including pneumonia. It is often linked to wearing contact lenses.[15]
Staphylococcus aureus and Methicillin-resistant *Staphylococcus aureus*	*S. aureus* infections are often acquired in hospital settings but can also be acquired elsewhere. They often affect skin and mucus membranes and can be drug resistant, as in the case of Methicillin-resistant *Staphylococcus aureus* (MRSA).[16]

THE RISE AND FALL OF THE ANTIBIOTIC AGE

Several years ago, the Canadian journalist Chris Wodskou stated that "a lot of medical and public health experts now fear that we're on the cusp of an unsettling new age . . . the Post-Antibiotic Age."[17] I believe that we are no longer living on the cusp, but have firmly moved and settled ourselves within this age.

In the second half of the twentieth century, antibiotics were dispensed almost as frequently as candy to knock out every form of bacterial illness, from UTIs to bacterial pneumonia, and many conditions in between. Countless people even went to their doctor demanding a prescription for antibiotic drugs for every cold or flu virus they encountered. Most doctors obliged these misinformed requests for drugs that kill bacteria, but offered no value in the face of viral illnesses, in an effort to appease their patients, placate their complaints, and to ensure their patients remained satisfied with their medical services. While many doctors may have believed the drugs would merely work as placebos, they didn't.

Pharmacists filled these prescriptions for antibiotic drugs, people popped them like candy, and urinated them into their toilets, the water from which eventually led to the water system. So, the patients who lacked even the most basic medical knowledge essentially dictated their treatment from the medical system from the doctors' offices to the pharmacies, simply by demanding an end to their uncomfortable, but usually mild, symptoms through the use of absolutely useless and ineffective drugs for viruses and the viral conditions they cause. Remember: *antibiotic* means "anti-bacterial," *not* "anti-viral."

And, in every place that antibiotics or their residues made their way, they began to shape the bacteria they encountered. The bodies of everyone who took antibiotics—whether for their correct antibacterial use or as placebo drugs used to "quell" the symptoms of people with viruses—became living laboratories where bacteria learned how to resist and survive against some of our once best medicines (when correctly used). The result: a plethora of stronger, more resilient bacteria, and eventually, superbugs, along with a set of increasingly useless antibiotic drugs.

When we received prescriptions for antibiotics used to actually treat the bacteria for which the drugs were intended, we may have inadvertently also contributed to their misuse. We may have taken them for a few days, but then stopped their use because we didn't feel better or our symptoms had not yet noticeably improved or subsided, incorrectly believing that they were not working. Or, we didn't take the drug for the full duration for which they were prescribed, or we missed doses due to our busy schedules. Doing any of these things may have actually given harmful bacteria an opportunity to learn how to outsmart, or resist, the drugs, contributing to the formation of superbugs within our own bodies.

At the same time, in a desperate attempt to capitalize on and profit from the antibacterial product fever that seemed to be sweeping the world, corporations began manufacturing and selling antibacterial everything, including: soaps, cleaning products, air "fresheners" or "disinfectants," "disinfecting wipes," "plug-ins," and more, scarring the commercial landscape with largely ineffective, chemical-saturated products. These products may have killed some of the bacteria they encountered but also left a wasteland of homes, offices, and land-fills full of bacteria that learned to surmount these toxic substances, once again, resulting in still more superbugs, and human and animal immune systems reduced by their exposure.

And, throughout the recent pandemic, we observed store after store carefully placing their bucket-sized pump bottle of hand sanitizer on a special table at the front of their store, café, or restaurant for every patron who entered to sanitize their hands. Little, if any, consideration was given to the harmful immune-damaging or immune-suppressing chemicals that might also be present in the products and penetrating the skin's surface to gain access to the bloodstream, or even whether the so-called active ingredients found in the products might be antibacte-rial but offer no value against viruses. Of course, there may have also been excellent natural products that have antiviral properties without the immune-suppressant effects of toxic ingredients, but it is unclear how many of the products on the market would fall into this category. It's likely small in contrast to the toxic varieties. Worse than that, in our desire to feel safe in the short-term, we may have further contributed to more superbugs in the coming years.

At the same time, veterinarians and factory farms also began mis-using antibiotics for pets and farm animals. By some estimates, at least half of all antibiotics used in the United States are used at large fac-tory farms[18] "to treat diseases spread by industrial husbandry practices, or simply to accelerate growth. As a result, farms have become giant Petri dishes for superbugs, especially multi-drug resistant *Staphylococcus aureus* or MRSA, which kills twenty thousand Americans every year—more than AIDS."[19]

Farms are not the only breeding grounds for drug-resistant bacteria; hospitals have also become hotbeds of resistant microbes. We frequently read about MRSA, C. diff, and carbapenem-resistant *Enterobacteriaceae* (CRE) infections that originate in hospital settings that can cause severe blood, colon, kidney, respiratory, and urinary tract conditions. In the case of CRE, these infections come from contaminated medical devices like catheters, ventilators, or surgical tools.[20]

Our collective germophobia and the resulting reliance on antibacterial consumer goods, combined with our mis-prescribing and misuse of antibiotic drugs, has led to the failing of what many people consider our best medicine against bacterial illnesses, and the resulting antibiotic resistance.

You may be wondering how all of these practices and activities can contribute to superbugs. Here are some of the ways in which bacteria outsmart antibiotics. By overcoming antibiotics, bacteria become stronger and may mutate to ensure their survival. So exactly how do they do this?

HOW DO BACTERIA BECOME SUPERBUGS?

Bacteria share resistance information, either directly, or by extruding it from their cells so that other bacteria can pick up the information at a later time. Here are three ways that bacteria share resistance information:

1. Encoding of plasmids, which are essentially DNA strands, to include resistance information that is then passed along to other bacteria. Because plasmids are highly mobile strands of genetic material, they are widely exchanged among bacteria.
2. Using "jumping genes," which are more often called transposons in the scientific world. These jumping genes allow bacteria to release a significant amount of resistance information into the environment where other bacteria can pick it up later.
3. Using viruses (yes, bacteria can use viruses!) known as bacteriophages, or bacterial viruses, that make copies of the components of genes that contain resistance information and then spread to other bacteria.[21]

It may shock you to know that the commonly used antibiotic drug known as tetracycline stimulates the transfer, mobilization, and movement of both plasmids and transposons by one hundred to one thousand times that of bacteria without exposure to the drug, even with low doses.[22] And, that's just one antibiotic drug, of which there are many in longstanding use over many years and currently in use today.

Don't forget that the common practice of flushing excess drugs down the toilet also sends these drugs into the water supply, as well as rivers, lakes, and other waterways, where bacteria living in these areas are exposed to the drugs on an ongoing basis. This ongoing exposure can drive their ability to learn resistance to the drugs. And, of course, the more we flush these drugs, or even just urinate those that our bodies haven't used, into the waterways, the more opportunity we give disease-causing bacteria to learn resistance to them and become superbugs.

While many believe that microbial resistance is inevitable, the reality is that drugs and excessive use of antibacterial products create resistance, but plant-based medicines do not. You'll learn more about that imminently.

It's less known how other types of infectious microbes become superbugs, but over time, it may become more evident.

OVERVIEW OF VIRUSES AND THEIR PRIMARY EFFECTS[23]

Virus Type	Primary Effects
Respiratory	Influenza viruses linked to the flu. Respiratory Syncytial Virus (RSV) linked to some colds, pneumonia, and bronchiolitis. Rhinovirus—most common virus linked to the common cold SARS-CoV-2 linked to Covid-19
Skin	Herpes Simplex I (HSV-I) linked to cold sores Varicella Zoster Virus (VZV) linked to chicken pox

OVERVIEW OF VIRUSES AND THEIR
PRIMARY EFFECTS (continued)

Virus Type	Primary Effects
Viral Food Poisoning	Hepatitis A impacts the liver Norovirus linked to gastrointestinal (GI) illness Rotavirus linked to diarrhea and dehydration
Sexually-Transmitted Illness (STIs)	Human Papillomavirus (HPV) Hepatitis B impacts the liver Herpes simplex-2 (HSV-2) linked to genital herpes Herpes Simplex-1 (HSV-1) can sometimes cause genital herpes Human Immunodeficiency Virus (HIV) affects some T-cells of the immune system
Other	Epstein-Barr Virus (EBV) is a type of herpes linked to mononucleosis (mono) West Nile Virus (WNV) commonly transmitted by mosquitoes, can cause fever and headaches, and in rare cases brain or spinal cord inflammation Enteroviruses are a group of viruses that can be linked to meningitis Cytomegaloviruses can cause cold sores or affect intestines, esophagus, lungs, brain, or nerves[24]

WHY YOU NEED TO SUPERCHARGE
YOUR IMMUNE SYSTEM

Whenever your immune system is functioning smoothly, you probably don't give it a second thought. When you start to feel a sore throat or fever, or notice that a wound has become infected, then you want to make sure your immune system can handle whatever infectious pathogen it has come into contact with.

While your immune system is powerful on its own, boosting it through the use of foods and natural medicines increases its ability to fight viruses, bacteria, and other foreign intruders that find their way into your body. You'll also reduce the chances of becoming ill, and if you do become sick, shorten the duration of the illness. But, perhaps the greatest advantage immune-boosting foods and natural medicines provide is their ability to improve your body's capacity to know when to fight without overreacting to intruders or attacking its own tissues. This enhanced intelligence of sorts is critical for your health and to reduce the likelihood of severe consequences of infectious diseases.

Now that you have a more thorough understanding of how your immune system functions, as well as why it needs your support, let me show you why natural medicines offer the best support.

BENEFITS OF COMPLEX NATURAL MEDICINES

Our ancestors' lengthy use of plant-based medicines over thousands of years contributed to our success on the planet today. We're alive because of their knowledge of plant medicines as well as their decisions to use medicines that work harmoniously with nature.

While I recognize that mushrooms are fungi and probiotics are bacteria and yeasts, and neither of them are plants, for the purpose of this book, I will include them among "plant medicines" or "plant-based medicines" to acknowledge that they are naturally occurring and not synthetic, laboratory-derived medicines like pharmaceutical drugs.

Did you know that most pharmaceutical drugs are easy targets for superbugs because they are chemically simplistic in their structures? It's true. Most pharmaceutical companies scour the Earth for new plant compounds that they can extract, synthesize, patent, and then manufacture into so-called wonder drugs that promise to reverse and even cure our worst ailments and diseases. But, in separating these plant compounds from the essential nutrients and other synergistic substances found naturally alongside the original compound, and then attempting to re-create these naturally occurring compounds in the laboratory, contrary to popular belief, they were frequently reducing the effectiveness of the plant medicine and creating drugs that carry long lists of side effects and, frequently, a steep price tag.

Pharmaceutical giants know the value of plant medicines. Otherwise, they wouldn't scour the Earth in search of the next great medicine from which to extract unique compounds—compounds that they'll later synthesize and patent. Most of these corporations hold patents on many once-natural but now synthetically derived drugs that allow them to charge sick people hundreds or even thousands of dollars each month, allowing them to profit to the tune of billions of dollars a year. But, that's a topic for another day. Plant medicines, by comparison, are largely affordable, and many are readily available.

Side effects from synthetic derivatives and profits from patents are just two of the issues linked to pharmaceutical drugs. They are usually made from one effective ingredient or compound along with many fillers, colors, and preservatives. Most bacteria, fungi, parasites, and viruses can overcome these simplistic medicines with relative ease. And, as you learned earlier, share this resistance information with other microbes to enable them to do the same. These simplistic medicines, along with their misuse or overuse has encouraged the proliferation of many superbugs.

By contrast, natural medicines, whether they are foods, herbs, essential oils, mushrooms, or some other natural substance, are far more chemically complex than their drug counterparts, making them very difficult for superbugs to outsmart. As a result, natural medicines do not cause resistance problems the way that drugs do.

Most herbal medicines and essential oils derived from them actually contain a hundred or more compounds. While our Western way of thinking has been shaped by the drug industry to consider that only one or a few of these compounds are actually "active ingredients," it is simply not the case. Some of the compounds may indeed stand out as superstars but, as in music, the lead instruments also need the rest of the orchestra to be complete; the same is true of the many compounds in herbal medicines. The many other vitamins, minerals, and phytonutrients (which literally means "plant nutrients") work synergistically to ensure the active ingredients are absorbed, work more effectively, and are less likely to cause harmful side effects.

These natural medicines also work more synergistically with the planet, reducing the likelihood of contributing to resistant bacteria, fungi, or viruses that, in turn, result in fewer serious or deadly infectious diseases with which we must contend.

Of course, natural medicines only work if they are used correctly, yet most people dabble in them like they are their latest hobby, without any consideration of the correct method of use. If they don't see immediate results, they assume the remedies didn't work and stop using them. As with anything, inappropriate use is a recipe for failure, not for success. If people took the same approach with synthetic drugs, the vast majority of them would be ruled out as ineffective simply because they don't provide immediate relief.

HOW TO CHOOSE YOUR NATURAL MEDICINES

While most natural remedies are highly effective and safe, there are some critical considerations to ensure their effectiveness and safe use.

Many of the natural remedies on the market are inferior quality and would be unlikely to yield any therapeutic benefit. It is important to choose high-quality nutritional supplements, herbs, essential oils, and other remedies to ensure you'll get great results if you use them correctly. Some products contain harmful ingredients that are best avoided, yet you won't find those ingredients listed on the label. Unfortunately, it is difficult to know a high-quality product from an inferior or dangerous one.

The realm of essential oils is particularly a free-for-all, as there are many poor-quality products on the market and many that are contaminated with fake ingredients, toxic solvents, and even cancer-causing phthalates. Many are diluted with similar-smelling, but cheaper, oils that will never yield the desired therapeutic effects because they aren't even the product you're trying to purchase. Avoid products labeled "fragrance" oils, "perfume" oils, or "natural identical" oils as they are usually synthetic and will not yield any therapeutic effects and may cause harmful reactions.

When it comes to natural remedies, like everything, you tend to get what you pay for, so if the price seems too good to be true, it probably is.

While it may seem like a good idea to choose organic products, the reality is that the term *organic* means different things in different countries, where many of the raw herbs are grown, so it may not mean anything.

When choosing plant-based medicines, be sure they are harvested in an environmentally sound way to avoid depleting important medicinal plants that may be nearing extinction or at risk of it if unscrupulous companies cause damage. For example, the essential oil copaiba is extracted from Amazon rainforest. Most companies cut down the trees to harvest the oil, but at least one company that I know of taps the trees like maple syrup during the time of year that it is safe to do so, and limits the amount of the resin they take from the tree to reduce its vulnerability to disease or likelihood of death. This may be difficult to discern as many companies make claims that are unsupported by their actions.

Choose products that are third-party laboratory tested since they are more likely to be transparent about their ingredients and purity.

If you are pregnant or lactating you should only use products that are proven safe during these times; unfortunately, many remedies have not been tested under these circumstances, for ethical reasons. As a result, there is insufficient safety testing for such uses and they may be best to avoid unless you have the approval of your physician or a qualified natural health professional.

Store your natural remedies, including nutritional supplements, herbs, and essential oils, in a dark place away from heat, light, and children.

Since it can take years to identify quality products, I've included some of my preferred products from my decades of experience on my website DrMichelleCook.com to help people make wise choices.

Do not discontinue any prescription medications without first consulting your doctor. And remember that herbs, essential oils, and nutritional supplements are natural medicines in their own right and therefore should not be mixed with synthetic medications without prior consultation with a knowledgeable health practitioner. While it's good to run them past your doctor, don't be surprised if she or he doesn't approve of the use of natural medicines. Most medical doctors have never taken a single course on natural medicines and are therefore unable to instruct their patients accordingly or provide accurate information in this regard. However, it is still best to inform them of all products you wish to use to prevent unwanted health implications or complications from drug- and plant-based medicines interacting.

It's important to remember that many natural herbs and the remedies derived from them have an exceptionally lengthy history of safe use—thousands of years in most cases. The fact that you exist on the planet at this time is a testament to the effectiveness of many natural remedies and their use among your ancient and more recent ancestors. It's worth considering them to give your immune system a boost and to help your body overcome harmful infectious illnesses. Whether you're interested in this book for prevention purposes or to help deal with a pre-existing ailment, there are many remedies that may be helpful.

2
Foods and Nutrients

Super-Powered Nutrition to Boost Your Immunity

The foods you eat and the beverages you drink become the cells that fashion your tissues, organs, and organ systems. The best way to transform your health and supercharge your immunity is to give your body optimal fuel that builds and nourishes healthy cells and improves the digestion, absorption, and assimilation of the food and beverages you consume.

When you eat, the foods and beverages you consume break down through digestion into their component nutrients: water, fiber, amino acids, essential fats, sugars, vitamins, minerals, phytonutrients (plant nutrients), and others. Your body transports these building blocks in the blood to the places they are needed to make them into healthy new cells, tissues, organs, and organ systems. So, it may come as no surprise to learn that if you want healthy immunity, you need to give your body the nutrition it needs to build healthy cells, which in turn become healthy bodily systems.

NUTRIENTS THAT BUILD
SUPERIOR IMMUNITY

Before we discuss the best nutrient-rich foods to feed your body, let's explore the nutrients that support healthy immunity. While all vitamins and most minerals are needed to ensure a strong immune system, some vitamins, minerals, and phytonutrients are especially critical for healthy immunity. The importance of vitamins is actually stated within the word itself. The word *vitamin* actually means "necessary for life." Derived from the words *vita,* meaning "life," and *amine,* meaning "a nitrogenous substance that is necessary for life,"[1] vitamins literally are essential for life. You cannot live without them. That's why I chuckle when I hear uninformed people say they don't believe that vitamins work. Not only do they work, they're keeping you alive as you make that false assertion, if you're among those doing so.

Certain nutrients are also integral to immunity because they help your body target and overcome infectious disease-causing microbes like bacteria, fungi, and viruses.

Rather than divide the nutrients by classifications (vitamins, minerals, and phytonutrients), you'll find them in alphabetical order. That way, you won't have to know how a nutrient is classified by scientists or nutritionists to find it within this chapter. For example, if you're wondering about quercetin, which has gotten a lot of media attention in recent years for its antiviral activity, you don't have to know that it is a phytonutrient to find information about it in this chapter. Simply search in alphabetical order through the nutrients below and you'll find quercetin slotted in exactly where you'd expect to find a nutrient beginning with the letter *Q*—after Omega-3 Fatty Acids and before Selenium.

In this chapter, you'll discover powerful immune-boosting and microbe-destroying nutrients that include: berberine, curcumin, epigallocatechin gallate (EGCG), glutathione, magnesium, N-acetyl cysteine, quercetin, selenium, vitamin C, and vitamin D. As discussed earlier, an argument could be made for inclusion of every nutrient, but that would take at least a full book-length work on its own, which is beyond the scope of this chapter, so you'll find those I've deemed most beneficial from my decades as a nutritionist.

While I've attempted to include research on the antibacterial, antifungal, and antiviral effects of these key nutrients, in some cases little research has been done, so, rather than mention it in every instance, the section is omitted. For example, little research has been done on the antifungal effects of N-acetyl cysteine so you'll only find the nutrients' antibacterial and antiviral benefits mentioned. That doesn't necessarily mean that the nutrient won't work against fungal infections, only that there is insufficient research to warrant its potential antifungal capacity within this chapter.

Let's begin our exploration of powerful nutrients and the foods or plants in which they are found.

Berberine—The Plant Nutrient That Packs a Punch Against Bacteria, Fungi, and Viruses Alike

Berberine is a phytonutrient extracted from plants like barberry, Oregon grape, and blue cohosh, among others, many of which are used in herbal medicine.[2] It is also found in a traditional Chinese medicine formula with a long history of use in the treatment of a wide range of conditions.[3] While few people have heard of this powerful nutrient, a growing body of research shows that it packs a punch against many different microbes, including bacteria, fungi, and viruses alike.

Research published in the medical journal *Frontiers of Medicine* found that berberine is antibacterial against *E. coli*.[4] Another study showed that berberine has antibacterial activity against a broad spectrum of bacterial varieties, including strains that are drug resistant.[5]

Berberine also demonstrates significant effectiveness against fungal infections like various strains of *Candida,* including against the biofilms they create. Biofilms are slimy coatings that bacteria create to protect themselves and reduce the likelihood of being detected and killed by the human immune system. In a study published in the journal

Drug Design, Development and Therapy, researchers found that berberine was highly effective at reducing all five of the *Candida* strains
they tested it against, as well as at inhibiting the biofilms they create.
Impressed by the significant antifungal effects of berberine, the scientists concluded, "Berberine might have novel therapeutic potential as
an antifungal agent or a major active component of antifungal drugs."[6]

Exciting research published in the *Archives of Virology* found that it
demonstrated antiviral activity on many viruses, including herpes simplex, human cytomegalovirus (HCMV), HPV, and HIV.[7]

Consult the At-a-Glance Nutrient Dosages Chart on pages 46–47
for dosage information on berberine.

Curcumin—Follow the Yellow Pigment Road to Stop Microbes in Their Tracks

Curcumin is one of a set of plant compounds known as curcuminoids
that are extracted from the yellow spice that gives curries their characteristic yellow color—turmeric. According to research published in the
journal *BioMed Research International,* researchers found that the plant
pigment demonstrated potent antibacterial, antifungal, and antiviral
activity,[8] making it an excellent choice in the prevention and treatment
of infectious diseases.

Curcumin demonstrated antibacterial activity against *S. aureus*
and *E. coli* when used in skin gels and applied to wounds.[9] It also
showed effectiveness against antibiotic-resistant MRSA when used
in conjunction with certain antibiotic drugs and even increased the
potency of the drugs, making them more effective against the drug-
resistant *Staphylococcus* infections, according to research in the journal
Phytomedicine.[10] Even when antibiotics weren't used alongside curcumin,
it demonstrated effectiveness against the two dozen other bacteria it was
tested against,[11] making it an excellent choice to address bacteria-caused
infections. Among bacteria tested, curcumin demonstrated effectiveness
against the frequently drug-resistant *H. pylori,*[12] which is often implicated in ulcers and gastrointestinal health issues.

Fungi have also demonstrated resistance against antifungal medications so finding natural remedies that can be used against them is critical to our health. Fortunately, curcumin demonstrated potent antifungal activity against a range of fungi, including *Candida albicans* (*C. albicans*), the fungus behind "yeast" infections. A bit of a misnomer, *C. albicans* is actually a fungus, not a yeast, that is linked to both intestinal and vaginal yeast infections. Curcumin was even effective against a range of *Candida* strains that are resistant to the drug fluconazole.[13]

Curcumin showed effectiveness against multiple strains of flu viruses and was also effective against respiratory syncytial virus (RSV), herpes simplex 1, and herpes simplex 2, the latter of which was effective when used vaginally.[14] Curcumin was found in a study published in *Phytotherapy Research* to inhibit the SARS-CoV-2 virus's ability to enter the cells, which viruses need to do to replicate and survive. It has also been found to reduce the sometimes-fatal cytokine storms that are linked to viral infections like serious cases of Covid-19.[15]

Consult the At-a-Glance Nutrient Dosages Chart on pages 46–47 for dosage information on curcumin.

Epigallocatechin Gallate (EGCG)— The Little Tea Nutrient That Could

You've probably heard about the incredible healing abilities of green tea, but few people know that, in addition to its heart-healing and anticancer properties, green tea and the potent compound found in it— epigallocatechin gallate (EGCG)—is also highly anti-infectious.

One of the primary phytonutrients found in green tea, EGCG has been identified in research as having antibacterial properties, on its own or in combination with antibiotics to bolster the drugs' effects, including against *S. aureus* and many other bacteria.[16] Other research in the *Journal of Applied Oral Science* is exploring the addition of EGCG into dental fillings since it has been found to inhibit some *Streptococcus* bacteria.[17] The same research also showed that EGCG demonstrates antifungal activity.[18]

Another study published in the *British Journal of Pharmacology* found that EGCG demonstrated antiviral activity on multiple families of viruses, including HIV, influenza A, and hepatitis C, and interfered with the viral replication process that is needed for survival of hepatitis B, herpes simplex, and adenoviruses.[19] Other research in the journal *Experimental and Therapeutic Medicine* found that EGCG blocked flu viruses from replicating[20]—a key process in the survival of viruses.

One cup (250 milliliters) of brewed green tea contains 50 to 100 milligrams of EGCG.[21] Consult the At-a-Glance Nutrient Dosages Chart on pages 46–47 for dosage information on EGCG.

Glutathione—The Missing Nutritional Link That Could Save Lives

One of the most powerful things you can do to boost your immune system and aid its ability to fight off infectious intruders is also one of the least known. Many people have not even heard of the nutrient glutathione, which is one of nature's greatest treasures when it comes to fighting disease-causing microbes. Glutathione is an antioxidant nutrient that is produced in the cells of your body, primarily from three building blocks of proteins called amino acids, including cysteine, glutamine, and glycine.[22]

Even moderate changes in glutathione levels in the body have a profound effect on the status of lymphocyte functions. You may recall from our earlier discussion that lymphocytes are the immune cells, known as natural killer cells, B cells and T cells, that attack invading bacteria, viruses, and other microbes.[23] What's more, the levels of this nutrient in your body could determine whether you have severe complications from an infection, and even whether you might live or die.

You might think that such an important, research-supported nutrient would be found in the medicine bag of every physician, yet most medical doctors have never heard of the nutrient, or ever studied it in school, and certainly do not prescribe it to their patients. Fortunately, a growing body of research brought this nutrient to the forefront of natural approaches to bacteria, viruses, and other conditions linked to harmful microbes, which may alert doctors to the importance of this readily available nutrient.

Research in the *International Journal of Medical Microbiology* found that glutathione on its own or in combination with antibiotic drugs may be effective in treating some bacterial infections, namely *A. baumanni,*[24] an opportunistic microbe that often impacts people who are immunocompromised, particularly as skin or respiratory infections, and is frequently drug resistant.[25] Other research found that glutathione was effective against *P. aeruginosa* and also boosted the effects of the antibiotic drug tetracycline against the bacteria.[26]

Glutathione has been discovered as the potential missing link in the prevention and treatment of serious viral-related complications. According to research in the medical journal *ACS Infectious Diseases,* a deficiency in the nutrient known as glutathione may be the cause of severe complications or death due to Covid-19.[27] Another study published in the *European Review for Medical and Pharmacological Sciences* confirmed the findings that a glutathione deficiency may play a central role in severe disease symptoms and death linked to Covid-19.[28]

Earlier research in the journal *Biological Chemistry* may provide the answers as to why glutathione may provide protection against viruses (and as this study also showed, against infectious bacteria as well). The researchers found that glutathione regulated the immune response, which not only helps the body attack foreign invaders like pathogens, it also prevents the immune system from overreacting to produce cytokine storms, which are potentially life-threatening inflammatory conditions.[29]

Many people, doctors included, assume that nutrients, herbs, and other natural medicines work similarly to drugs in that they tend to perform one function. As a result, I've had countless patients tell me that their doctors told them they shouldn't use anything that boosts immunity if they have an autoimmune condition—conditions in which the body cannot properly differentiate foreign invaders from its own tissues and attacks its own tissues—such as Addison's disease, Hashimoto's thyroiditis, inflammatory bowel disease (IBD), lupus erythematosus, multiple sclerosis, and rheumatoid arthritis, among others. Drugs tend to be one or two compounds that perform one or a couple of functions, such as target bacteria or viruses (different drugs). Nutrients and herbs tend to be much more chemically complex and are actually much smarter. The same nutrient that boosts immunity when needed may also reduce immune system overactivity when needed. That's the case with glutathione.

For those suffering from autoimmune conditions, glutathione is particularly beneficial. Research published in the journal *Autoimmunity Reviews* found that glutathione intake helped to regulate the body's immune response.[30]

Poor nutrition, aging, stress, and exposure to environmental and food toxins cause glutathione levels to wane over time. Additionally, lack of sleep or insomnia may contribute to reduced glutathione levels in the body.[31]

Glutathione is found in foods like asparagus and avocado, as well as other freshly-picked fruits and vegetables. Additionally, consuming the following foods may be helpful for your body to manufacture glutathione as they contain some of the building blocks needed for glutathione production: bok choy, broccoli, Brussels sprouts, cauliflower, chicken, eggs, fish, flaxseed, garlic, legumes, milk thistle (an herb), nuts, onions, and a type of seaweed known as *guso*.[32]

Food sources will be beneficial but may not provide the amount of glutathione needed to address serious infectious diseases. Supplements may be necessary, but most glutathione supplements simply do not absorb well, so you're basically throwing your money away to purchase them. As a result, I have not included dosage information for glutathione supplements in the At-a-Glance Nutrient Dosages Chart on pages 46–47. After many years of searching, I found a liquid glutathione supplement that seems to absorb well and that I've personally used with great success, and all the people I've recommended it to have also reported improved energy, immunity, and overall feelings of wellness when using it. I share the information for the glutathione product on my website DrMichelleCook.com.

Two Vitamins That Help Prevent the Spread of the Human Papilloma Virus

A team of scientists led by C. J. Piyathilake of the Department of Nutrition Sciences at the University of Alabama at Birmingham attempted to determine whether supplementation with folate (vitamin B9) and vitamin B12 would have an effect on HPV and cervical cancer linked to this virus among women.

They attempted to identify any associations between serum concentrations of folate and vitamin B12 and high-risk HPV infections by evaluating 724 women in a screening study in the state of Andhra Pradesh, India.

They found that women with the highest concentrations of serum folate and vitamin B12 had the lowest risk of being positive for high-risk HPVs compared to those with lower blood levels of folate and vitamin B12.

The scientists published their results in the *International Journal of Women's Health* and concluded that: "These results demonstrated that improving folate and vitamin B12 status in Indian women may have a beneficial impact on the prevention of cervical cancer. Micronutrient based interventions for control of high-risk HPV infections may represent feasible alternatives to vaccine based approaches to HPV disease prevention."[33]

Considering the controversy surrounding HPV vaccines and the likelihood that their results with Indian women are applicable to other women, the results suggest that supplementation with folate and vitamin B12 (or a single B-complex vitamin that includes both folate and B12) may help prevent HPV and cervical cancer.

Note that folic acid is the synthetic form of folate.

Magnesium—The Mineral That Unlocks Vitamin D's Antimicrobial Potency

Magnesium may not be one of the primary antiviral nutrients that comes to mind but magnesium regulates antiviral immunity, according to research in *Nature Reviews: Immunology*.[34] And research also shows that adequate levels of magnesium are needed to activate vitamin D.[35] Considering the essential nature of vitamin D to protect against viral infections like Covid-19 and others, I would be remiss if I didn't include magnesium among the nutrients that are needed to boost immunity and fight infectious diseases.

According to research published in the medical journal *Open Heart,* researchers found that "the vast majority of people in modern societies are at risk for magnesium deficiency."[36] Such a mineral deficiency leaves people vulnerable for vitamin D deficiency, which as you'll learn momentarily can be potentially serious, particularly where infectious diseases are concerned. Blood magnesium tests are not the best way to determine magnesium status.[37] In cases where magnesium deficiency is present,[38] supplementation is worth considering.

Consult the At-a-Glance Nutrient Dosages Chart on pages 46–47 for dosage information on magnesium.

N-acetyl Cysteine (NAC)— The Infection-Blocking Nutrient

N-acetyl Cysteine (NAC) is one of the key nutrients needed by your body to make glutathione, which we discussed earlier. Boosting your intake of this nutrient may help your body make more of the critical antioxidant and anti-infectious glutathione. Additionally, research shows that NAC may also help address bacterial infections and their protective biofilms that can make the infections hard for the immune system to tackle.

According to research in the medical journal *BMC Microbiology,* N-acetyl cysteine demonstrates potent antibacterial effects against a group of bacteria known as mycobacteria.[39] There are many species of bacteria collectively known as mycobacteria, some of which have been linked to conditions like leprosy and tuberculosis.[40] Researchers of the *BMC Microbiology* study determined that NAC "may limit *M. tuberculosis* infection and disease both through suppression (of a person's immune response) and through direct antimicrobial activity."[41] Additionally, when used in conjunction with antibiotics, researchers have shown that NAC works to break down biofilms, allowing the nutrient-drug combination to overcome bacteria that are resistant to drugs alone.[42] Other research suggests that NAC may hold promise in the treatment of tuberculosis. This is welcome news considering that *Mycobacterium tuberculosis* (*M. tuberculosis*) is showing a greater rate of drug resistance.[43]

Research shows that this antioxidant nutrient, which boosts glutathione levels in the body,[44] may block the penetration of the SARS-CoV-2 virus into the cells, which researchers indicate is likely to attenuate the risk of developing Covid-19.[45] In another study published in the medical journal *Antiviral Research,* scientists found that NAC suppressed the ability of the Coxsackie B virus to replicate while also quelling inflammation that can be linked to viral disease complications.[46]

Consult the At-a-Glance Nutrient Dosages Chart on pages 46–47 for dosage information on NAC.

Omega-3 Fatty Acids—Immune-Boosters That Help Block Sometimes Deadly Cytokine Storms

Eating more healthy fats known as Omega-3s or Omega-3 fatty acids could save your life. Powerful natural anti-inflammatories, Omega-3 fatty acids are well-known for their ability to quell inflammation, but research published in the medical journal *BMJ Nutrition, Prevention & Health* found that they could also control frequently deadly immune reactions known as cytokine storms. When a severe infection attacks the respiratory system, it can lead to a condition called acute respiratory distress syndrome (ARDS), which is characterized by excessive and damaging inflammation known as a cytokine storm.[47]

You may recall hearing about cytokine storms in our dealings with the Covid-19 pandemic, since they were behind some of the fatalities linked with the viral condition.

It's a good idea to become more aware of the types of fats you're eating on a regular basis as they can be contributing to your immune health or lack thereof. Most people eat a large amount of Omega-6 fatty acids, which throws off the ratio of Omega-6 to Omega-3 fatty acids in favor of inflammation in the body, which can leave your immune and respiratory systems vulnerable to inflammation, like that caused by cytokine storms. The ratio should be one to one or two to one Omega-6 to Omega-3, but most people eat them in a forty to one ratio, meaning they are consuming far more Omega-6 fatty acids than they should be getting, which is likely leaving them at risk for inflammation.

Omega-6 fatty acids are found in most foods that contain corn, sunflower, and safflower oils (which include "vegetable oils") as well as from eating the meat of animals that eat a diet high in these fats. Most prepared, processed, and packaged foods, as well as restaurant and take-out foods, are high in these oils. Baked goods are also usually high in these oils as they are primarily made from butter, margarine, and vegetable oil. High protein diets also tend to throw off the balance of the Omega-6 to Omega-3 ratio. Ideally, reduce your intake of these foods while increasing your intake of Omega-3-rich foods.

Omega-3 fatty acids are primarily found in the oils of cold-water fish, such as salmon, mackerel, herring, sardines, and anchovies, as well as nuts and seeds like flax, hemp, and walnut. Add flax oil or flaxseeds to your salad dressings, organic popcorn, oatmeal, smoothies, or other foods on a daily basis for best results.

Quercetin—The Plant Nutrient That Kicks Viruses to the Curb

Quercetin is a plant pigment (known as a flavonoid) that is found in apples, asparagus, black currants, blueberries, broccoli, cranberries, green peppers, green tea, onions, raspberries, red leaf lettuce, strawberries, and tomatoes.[48,49]

Quercetin's antiviral properties have been the subject of numerous studies.[50] One study published in the medical journal *Viruses* found that quercetin inhibited a wide spectrum of flu viruses' ability to enter the cells,[51] which they need to do for their survival.[52] The nutrient has demonstrated effectiveness against viruses on its own or in combination with other treatments. Because both quercetin and vitamin C have antiviral and immune-regulating properties, they work synergistically to improve the effectiveness of each natural remedy against viruses like SARS-CoV-2—the virus behind Covid-19. Additionally, vitamin C recycles quercetin, thereby increasing its efficacy.[53]

Quercetin has been shown to inhibit respiratory viruses in cell studies, including inhibiting rhinoviruses, coxsackie viruses, and polio viruses. It demonstrates beneficial effects against RSV, polio viruses, herpes simplex viruses, and cytomegalovirus. Its effects have been linked to the nutrient's ability to block viral entry or inhibit their ability to replicate.[54]

Consult the At-a-Glance Nutrient Dosages Chart on pages 46–47 for dosage information on quercetin.

Selenium—The Mineral That Reduces Susceptibility to Viruses

Selenium is an essential mineral needed for many functions in the body, including the maintenance of a healthy immune system. While many nutrients are needed in supporting roles for healthy immunity, selenium (along with zinc) play leading roles when it comes to defending the body against bacterial and viral infections.[55]

A deficiency in the mineral selenium is linked to a higher susceptibility to higher RNA viral infections as well as more severe illness.[56] Since viruses are particles of genetic material, they are classified as either DNA or RNA.[57] In a study published in the journal *Nutrients,* scientists recommended supplementation with selenium (as well as vitamin D and zinc) in high-risk areas and among high-risk populations for Covid-19, and as soon as possible after someone contracts Covid-19.[58]

Foods highest in selenium include: pork, beef, turkey, chicken, fish, eggs, yogurt, shellfish, beef, turkey, chicken, eggs, brown rice, sunflower seeds, baked beans, mushrooms, oatmeal, spinach, yogurt, lentils, cashews, and bananas.[59]

Consult the At-a-Glance Nutrient Dosages Chart on pages 46–47 for dosage information on selenium.

Vitamin C—The Most Overlooked and Misused Vitamin

Almost everyone knows about vitamin C and takes it at the first sign of a cold, but few people know just how powerful this vitamin is. Vitamin C, or ascorbic acid as it is technically known, is an essential vitamin with well-established antimicrobial properties.[60] It works on many levels to support your immune system health and to overcome infectious disease, including: (1) supporting lymphocyte activity, (2) increasing interferon-a production, (3) modulating cytokines, (4) reducing inflammation, (5) improving endothelial dysfunction, and (6) restoring mitochondrial function.[61]

Additionally, exciting research published in *Frontiers in Immunology* shows it has a synergistic antiviral effect when combined with quercetin in the prevention and treatment of SARS-CoV-2 infections.[62] In other words, the two nutrients were found to be more powerful when used simultaneously. Additionally, as you learned earlier, it works synergistically with quercetin and has the ability to recycle quercetin so it remains intact and effective longer than it otherwise would.[63]

Vitamin C is found in tomatoes, red peppers, lemons, oranges, grapefruit, limes, pomegranates, strawberries, black currants, spinach, beet greens, tomatoes, sprouts, and red peppers.

While food sources are essential and I encourage you to ensure their inclusion in your diet on a regular basis, if you're suffering from an infection, you may need more vitamin C than food alone can provide. And, before you mention that 100-milligram or 500-milligram vitamin C pill you're taking, or the amount you're getting in your multivitamin pill, I think it's important to mention that this is only a place to start, in terms of using vitamin C against infections. However, most people simply aren't using vitamin C correctly to derive its impressive anti-infectious benefits.

In my clinical and personal experience, high doses of vitamin C have powerful effects against bacterial or viral infections. By high doses, I'm referring to 2,000 milligrams taken every two to three hours at the first sign of an infection, up to about 10,000 milligrams daily for short-term periods like a few days or while dealing with an acute infection.

That amount greatly exceeds the recommended daily intake amount so you should only do so with your doctor's approval and for the short-term. But I can share that I've used this protocol personally and with many people over the years with great success at knocking out an infection quickly and completely. I don't recommend taking more than about 2,000 milligrams daily after the infection has cleared or after about a week of higher dosages. Consult the At-a-Glance Nutrient Dosages Chart on pages 46–47 for dosage information on vitamin C.

Vitamin D—The King of Super-Powered Immunity Nutrients That May Save Your Life

As you have seen, there are many nutrients that are vital to healthy immunity, but arguably, none surpasses the importance of vitamin D (and possibly glutathione, which we discussed earlier). Not only is it one of the primary nutrients to support the immune system's healthy functioning, it is also one of the primary antiviral vitamins.

Did you know that supplementing with this affordable and readily available nutrient could reduce your risk of dying from a virus, and may even save your life?[64] Vitamin D reduces the risk of dying from Covid-19 by 370 percent! And that's not all. Research in the *Archives of Microbiology* stated: "According to our findings, 84.4% of patients with Covid-19 in this study had vitamin D deficiency." In other words, a vitamin D deficiency may have left people vulnerable to the virus, which means that correcting the deficiency may help prevent someone from getting it in the first place. The scientists found that vitamin D not only modulated the immune system but also inhibited the virus's ability to replicate.[65]

This critical nutrient helps to modulate the function of the immune system,[66] meaning increasing its function when necessary but also preventing it from overworking in the case of cytokine storms or autoimmune conditions. Vitamin D receptors are found in most of the cells of the immune system, including B and T lymphocytes, monocytes, and macrophages, among others.[67]

Yet, shockingly, estimates suggest that one billion[68] people worldwide suffer from this nutrient deficiency that puts them at risk of bacterial or viral threats and even an increased risk of death from these microbes.

Research in the journal *ACS Infectious Diseases* showed that vitamin D deficiency has been found among those with increased incidence of *Streptococcus* bacterial infections, which include skin and soft tissue infections, pneumonia, meningitis, sinusitis, otitis media (ear infections), sepsis (dangerous blood infections), and even death.[69]

A significant body of research also demonstrates vitamin D's antiviral properties. Multiple studies even show that vitamin D is so powerful that supplementation could significantly reduce severe complications linked to the SARS-CoV-2 virus and even reduce the risk of death.[70,71,72] Vitamin D has been shown to reduce viruses' ability to survive and replicate in the body, as well as reduce the highly inflammatory cytokine storms that are often linked to severe illness and death due to viruses, including Covid-19.[73] Additional research published in the journal *Nutrients* found that vitamin D supplementation improved the survival rate among frail, elderly Covid-19 patients.[74]

A typical dose is 2,000 to 4,000 international units (IU) of vitamin D3 (cholecalciferol) or synthetic vitamin D2 for vegans.[75] Moderate sunlight exposure directly on skin devoid of sunscreen is a source of vitamin D but it is best not to wash the sun-kissed area for several hours afterward. Food sources for Vitamin D include fish, fish oil, sweet potatoes, sunflower seeds, mushrooms, and some sprouts.

Even those who supplement with this vitamin rarely take the correct form of the vitamin, in high enough doses, for long enough periods of time to get these results. Make sure you're getting the correct form of vitamin D (cholecalciferol or vitamin D3) for three to four months to eliminate the deficiency that plagues approximately 50 percent of the population.[76] Because vitamin D does *not* work properly without at least 400 milligrams of magnesium daily to activate vitamin D's immune-boosting effects, it is best to consider a magnesium supplement along with your Vitamin D.

Zinc—The Critical Mineral for Super-Powered Immunity

Zinc is an essential mineral needed for many functions in your body, including a healthy immune system.

Because zinc is involved in many pathways involving microbes in the body, it has the potential to be a novel strategy in the prevention or treatment of infectious disease conditions.[77] Zinc has been found beneficial in the treatment of drug-resistant bacterial infections, according to research published in the journal *Applied Microbiology and Biotechnology*.[78] Research in the *Turkish Journal of Gastroenterology* found that zinc supplementation reduced the duration of suffering of children with diarrhea resulting from microbial infections.[79]

Zinc has an important role to play in the prevention and treatment of fungal diseases. In a study published in the *Journal of Clinical Biochemistry and Nutrition,* researchers found that children in intensive care who were vulnerable to drug-resistant *Candida* fungal infections had a reduced incidence of fungal infections and the disease symptoms they create. They also had shorter stays in intensive care units and even a reduced incidence of death.[80]

There is an abundance of scientific evidence to support the use of zinc in the treatment of viral conditions, including the common cold and herpes simplex viruses.[81] When zinc lozenges or syrup is taken within twenty-four hours of the first symptoms of a cold, it can reduce the duration of the cold.[82] Zinc plays a critical role in the protection of the tissues in the respiratory tract, preventing the ability of viruses to enter as well as to ensure a balanced function of the immune system. It is considered probable that zinc status may be one of the factors predisposing people to infection or complications with Covid-19.[83] Zinc plays such a critical role in ensuring our immunity to viruses that zinc-deficient populations have even been found to be at a greater susceptibility to HIV and hepatitis C viruses.[84]

Zinc is found in chicken and red meat, as well as many vegetarian sources, which include pumpkin seeds, sunflower seeds, seafood, whole grains and whole grain bread, sprouts, soybeans, onions, beets or beet greens, carrots, peas, dark leafy green vegetables, nuts and nut butters (especially Brazil nuts), and legumes (black beans, chickpeas, kidney beans, navy beans, pinto beans, Romano beans, etc.). It is also a good idea to eat fermented foods as well since zinc tends to become more bioavailable during the fermentation process. These foods include miso, tempeh, sourdough breads, fermented vegetables, seed and nut cheeses that are fermented, and non-dairy yogurt.

Avoid intra-nasal zinc as it has been linked to a loss of smell.[85] Consult the At-a-Glance Nutrient Dosages Chart for dosage information on zinc.

AT-A-GLANCE NUTRIENT DOSAGES[86]

While obtaining nutrition from food is ideal, sometimes our bodies need higher amounts than is readily available in food, particularly to fight viruses.

Nutritional Supplement	Daily Dose
Berberine	1,500 mg daily up to 6 months[87]
Curcumin	3 g daily up to 3 months 8 g daily up to 2 months[88]
Epigallocatechin Gallate	338–704 mg[89]
Folate (Vitamin B9)	Choose folate rather than synthetic folic acid. 400 mcg daily[90]
Glutathione	Glutathione supplements vary greatly in their ability to be absorbed and most are minimally absorbed. I therefore do NOT recommend most glutathione supplements. See DrMichelleCook.com for more information and recommendations.

AT-A-GLANCE NUTRIENT DOSAGES (*continued*)

Nutritional Supplement	Daily Dose
Magnesium	Women age 19–30: 310 mg Women age 31+: 320 mg Men 19–30: 400 mg Men 31+: 420 mg[91]
N-acetyl Cysteine (NAC)	600–1200 mg[92]
Omega-3 Fatty Acids	Most Omega-3 fatty acid supplements are available as fish oil supplements: 1,000 mg 2 times daily Or as DHA-EPA (docosahexanoic acid, eicosapentanoic acid): 180 mg EPA and 120 mg DHA daily
Quercetin	1 g daily up to 12 weeks[93]
Selenium	55–400 mcg[94] Taking 400 mcg of selenium should only be used for acute purposes such as the onset of a virus but should not be continued for the long-term.
Vitamin B12	1,000 mcg daily[95]
Vitamin C	100–2,000 mg[96] Some nutritional practitioners recommend 2,000 mg every few hours during acute viral infections until bowel tolerance is reached (loose stools), then reduce the daily amount by 1,000 mg afterward. Do not exceed 2,000 mg in a single dose.*
Vitamin D	50–100 mcg/2,000–4,000 IU[97]
Zinc	Women: 8–40mg Men: 11–40mg[98] Avoid intra-nasal zinc

*Follow package instructions for the remedy you select. Do not exceed daily doses unless you are working with a qualified health practitioner. Some health professionals may advise higher doses to treat viral infections. Consult your physician if you have any health issues or are taking any medications.

Nutritional supplements can be highly beneficial to keep your immune system strong, hold viruses at bay, or to support your body while battling them.

Supporting Nutrients for Healthy
Immunity and Their Best Food Sources

There are many other important nutrients needed to ensure healthy immunity, most of which are possible to obtain in sufficient amounts through foods. These nutrients include:

Allicin: Allicin is a phytonutrient found in pungent foods like onions and garlic that is known for its antiviral compounds.

B-Complex Vitamins (especially Vitamin B6, folate [B9], and B12)[99]: B-complex vitamins are a group of vitamins that are needed to ensure many healthy functions in the body. Vitamin B6 is essential to maintain a healthy immune system and helps protect the respiratory tract from pollution and infection. Vitamin B6 is primarily found in carrots, apples, organ meats, bananas, leafy green vegetables, brown rice, root vegetables, strawberries, sweet potatoes, cantaloupe, kale, green vegetables, and beans. Folate is found in legumes, asparagus, eggs, beets, leafy greens, citrus fruits, Brussels sprouts, broccoli, nuts and seeds, beef liver, wheat germ, papaya, bananas, avocado, and fortified grains.[100] Vitamin B12 is found in dairy products, eggs, fish, meat, and poultry. Additionally, some vegan foods that may contain vitamin B12 include spirulina, other algae, barley grass, sprouts, nori, other types of seaweed, tempeh, fortified milk substitutes, other fortified packaged foods (meat substitutes and breakfast cereals), mushrooms, miso, fermented foods, and nutritional yeast. But, most of these sources are considered controversial because their vitamin B12 is not truly vitamin B12 but analogs that are believed to block absorption. The jury is still out on vitamin B12 food sources so it is best to supplement, particularly if you're vegan or vegetarian.

Carotenoids (Alpha carotene, Beta carotene, and Others): These are the immune-boosting phytonutrients that give foods their characteristic orange and green color. Carotenoids are found in apricots, broccoli, carrots, collards, leafy greens, kale, mangoes, melons, papayas, peaches, sweet potatoes, pumpkin, spinach, squash, and tomatoes. Carotenoids are a group of potent nutrients that can help to protect the lungs.

Copper: Copper plays an essential, albeit supporting, role in ensuring a healthy immune system.[101] Copper is found in liver, oysters, spirulina, shiitake mushrooms, nuts, seeds, lobster, leafy greens, and dark chocolate.[102]

Iron: Like copper, iron plays a supporting role in antibacterial and antiviral defense.[103] There are two types of iron: heme and non-heme. Many nutritionists advise people to obtain heme iron from meat sources such as red meat, liver, poultry, and fish, as they suggest it is better absorbed. While that may be partly true, red meat, organ meat, and poultry sources of iron typically contain excessive hormones, saturated fats, antibiotics, and other substances that may negate their value. Additionally, they don't contain vitamin C, which is also needed for iron absorption. Vegetarian (non-heme) sources of iron include prunes, raisins, figs, apricots, bananas, walnuts, kelp, beans, lentils, dark leafy greens, asparagus, and peaches. Incidentally, most of these foods also contain vitamin C, which helps with the absorption of iron in the body.

Terpene Limonoids: These are phytonutrients found in citrus fruit like grapefruit, lemons, limes, and oranges that have antiviral properties.

Vitamin A: Vitamin A, or its precursors, which are a group of nutrients collectively known as carotenoids (alpha-carotene, beta-carotene, lutein, zeaxanthin, etc.), are an anti-inflammatory vitamin that is essential to healthy immune function.[104]

Vitamin E: Vitamin E works as a powerful antioxidant that reduces the damage to the cells. It is found in eggs, whole grain breads and cereals, wheat germ, nuts, seeds, liver, unrefined vegetable oils, and dark green vegetables.

Top 9 Immune-Boosting Breakfast Ideas

We all know that breakfast is the most important meal of the day, and when it comes to strengthening your immune system, that has never been more accurate.

Before I share my picks for the top nine immune-boosting breakfasts, it is important to consider that what you eat is as important as what you don't eat. Skip the sugary donut, Danish, or breakfast cereals. Even a small amount of sugar can depress your immune system for as long as four to six hours. So regardless of which breakfast you choose, keep it low in sugars of all kinds—both refined and so-called "healthy" sweeteners, since they all have the same immune-lowering effect.

Here are some breakfast ideas to make your first meal of the day a powerhouse immune-booster:

Start with a Glass of Water with Lemon, Lime, or Grapefruit Juice: These juices are high in immune-boosting vitamin C and the antiviral phytonutrients called terpene limonoids that help give cold and flu viruses the boot.

Enjoy a Spanish Omelet or **Spanish Tofu Scramble:** Be sure to boost its healing properties by adding allicin-containing onions and garlic and vitamin-C-rich tomatoes and red peppers. Add a pinch or two of turmeric to give your tofu or eggs a brilliant yellow color while also adding an extra punch to any viruses you may have been in contact with.

Go for Granola: Most commercial granola is loaded with immune-suppressing sugar or high fructose corn syrup. Instead of these packaged options, make a simple immune-boosting granola from oats, flax seeds, sunflower seeds, pumpkin seeds, cinnamon, chopped almonds, a touch of honey or pure maple syrup (just a bit), and a little coconut oil or olive oil. Mix together and bake at 300 degrees until lightly browned (about ten to twenty minutes).

Allow to fully cool and store in an airtight container for up to a week. Eat on its own or add almond milk. The essential fats found in flax and pumpkin seeds are needed for a healthy immune system. Pumpkin seeds add a dose of zinc, which is also critical for immune health.

Savor a Sweet Potato Hash: Made with sweet potatoes, onions, garlic, red peppers, and beta-carotene- and vitamin B6-containing kale, sweet potato hash can give you important nutrients to build your immune system. Sweet potatoes contain vitamin B6, which is an important immune-system strengthener, along with beta carotene, the precursor of immune-building vitamin A, and even a vegetarian source of vitamin D, which reduces the risk of catching a cold or flu and speeds recovery.

Go for a Side of Grapefruit: This fruit is packed with vitamin C and antiflu phytonutrients known as terpene limonoids. These compounds are naturally antiviral, giving your immune system assistance to fight infection.

Brown Rice with Almond Milk and Cinnamon: Brown rice is a good source of vitamin B6, which protects the lungs against foreign invaders. Brown rice also contains the potent antioxidants vitamin E and zinc.

Cooked Quinoa or Oats with Apples: Protein-rich quinoa doesn't need to be reserved for lunch or dinner. Give it a breakfast twist by adding chopped apple during the cooking process. Alternatively, opt for oatmeal. Be sure to sprinkle cinnamon over your breakfast for an anti-infectious boost.

Go Green (Tea, That Is): There are dozens of reasons to drink green tea, but during the colder seasons or when you're trying to prevent or treat infections, there are even more. So, it's a great idea to finish off your immune-boosting breakfast with a hot cup of green tea sweetened with the herb stevia (to avoid immune crashes linked to sugar).

POTENT IMMUNE-BOOSTING FOODS
TO ADD TO YOUR DAILY DIET

You learned about many great immune-boosting foods, but there are a few that stand above the crowd. And, fortunately, they're delicious too, so keeping your immune system strong and healthy never tasted so good. Some of the best immune-boosting foods include:

Beets: Rich in the immune-boosting mineral zinc, beets, along with their leafy greens, are a great addition to your diet. Beets are also a rich source of prebiotics, the foods eaten by probiotics, or beneficial microbes, in your intestines, which help to balance your gut flora for even stronger immunity (see chapter 4). By eating more beets you'll feed the healthy bacteria and other beneficial microbes that give your gut and immune health a boost. You can also add them to fresh juice, grate and add them to salads and sandwiches, or roast and enjoy them on their own.

Blueberries: Blueberries don't just taste amazing they are packed with nutrients known as flavonoids that give them their gorgeous color and delicious taste. Research in the journal *Advances in Nutrition* shows that flavonoids, like those found in blueberries, boost the immune system.[105] Eat fresh blueberries on their own or atop salads or added to smoothies. Frozen blueberries that have been slightly thawed taste like blueberry sorbet and make a delicious dessert on their own.

Citrus Fruits: Grapefruit, lemons, limes, oranges, and other citrus fruit are excellent sources of immune-boosting vitamin C, making them great choices to include in your daily diet. Juice them or add them to salads or salad dressings, or in the case of grapefruit and oranges, eat them on their own as a quick snack.

Flaxseeds and Flaxseed Oil: Flaxseeds and flaxseed oil contain plentiful amounts of the essential fatty acids known as Omega-3 fatty acids that give your immune system a boost and help to keep it functioning well on a regular basis. Add flaxseeds or oil to your smoothie or top previously-cooked vegetables with a splash of flax oil and sea salt.

Garlic and Onions: Rich in immune-boosting allicin, garlic helps to stave off colds and flu by giving your immune system a boost. Cooking reduces the potency of garlic but both cooked and raw garlic are still worth eating on a daily basis. Add some garlic to your soups, stews, chili, and, of course, combined with chickpeas, lemon juice, tahini, olive oil, and a touch of salt for a delicious hummus.

Kefir: A beverage similar to yogurt but thinner, kefir comes from the Turkish word *keif,* which means "good feeling" probably because, let's face it, we feel better when we're not sick. Kefir offers immune-boosting health benefits due to its many different strains of beneficial bacteria and yeasts.[106] Make sure the one you choose contains "live cultures."

Kimchi: The national dish of Korea, kimchi is a spicy condiment that has been found in research published in the *Journal of Medicinal Food* to offer immune-boosting benefits.[107]

Manuka Honey: Research published in the journal *Archives of Medical Research* found that manuka honey has excellent inhibitory effects against the flu.[108]

Pumpkin Seeds: Pumpkin seeds contain plentiful amounts of the immune-boosting fats known as Omega-3 fatty acids, along with the essential immune health mineral zinc, making them an excellent choice to include in your diet. Throw them on top of your salads, grind them and add them to flour for baking, or snack on them as is.

Walnuts: Raw, unsalted walnuts are rich sources of immune-boosting Omega-3 fatty acids. If you don't like the taste of walnuts, I urge you to try ones that are raw, unsalted, and kept in the refrigerator section of your health food store since they are typically fresher than the ones found in packages in the center aisles of the grocery store. The bitter taste most people attribute to walnuts is actually a sign that they have gone rancid. Fresh walnuts have a buttery and delicious taste.

Yogurt: Yogurt and vegan yogurt contain beneficial bacteria that boost your gut health, which in turn, boost your immune system health. Make sure the yogurt you select contains "live cultures." Learn how to make your own dairy-free yogurt with probiotics in my book, *The Cultured Cook*.

Eating a healthy diet replete with the foods that support optimal immunity is as easy as incorporating more of the foods mentioned above and supplementing with key nutrients that build super-powered immunity.

3

Herbs and Essential Oils

All-Star Immune Boosters

Our heavy reliance on drugs to address whatever ails us, from headaches and indigestion to more serious health concerns like infections or cancer, have led us to believe that drugs are our best weapon against diseases of all kinds, including in our battle against bacteria, fungi, viruses, or other microbes. The massive advertising budgets of multi-billion-dollar pharmaceutical corporations and the ads we see on television, hear on radio, view on websites, and see in magazines and newspapers perpetuate this belief. At every turn, we see another ad for symptoms from which we may be suffering, along with what appears to be a solution at the drop of a pill, along with a glassful of water to push it down.

While herbs lay humbly upon the ground barely noticed and largely unrecognizable to most people, and lack the marketing boards or massive budgets of their synthetic drug counterparts, they are powerful natural medicines that are far more potent than most people realize.

Many herbs have been on the planet for thousands of years with a history of safe and effective use by our ancestors throughout that time. Compare that to the less than two-hundred-year history of pharmaceutical drugs (typically much less than that, and often only a handful of years), most of which have voluminous lists of harmful, and even sometimes deadly, side effects.

Fortunately, a growing body of research supports the use of herbal medicines, justifying their effective use for thousands of years by our ancestors. In this chapter, we'll explore the many powerful immune-boosting herbs. Most herbs have some degree of effectiveness against bacteria, viruses, and other microbes, and indeed whole volumes could be written on the topic, so it is difficult to narrow the list to just the most effective ones. And, as we gain constantly evolving insight through research into the medicinal properties of herbal medicines, today's choice might be different tomorrow; however, the herbs I've included have a lengthy history of use to accompany the research that supports their use.

GETTING STARTED IN HERBAL MEDICINE

We'll discuss the various herbal remedies momentarily, but there are some herbal fundamentals to consider before doing so, or before you head to your local health food store, online herbal apothecary, or to your local herbal product purveyor. It's important to understand the strengths and weaknesses of the various forms of herbal preparation to help you determine which might be best suited to deal with infectious conditions or your specific condition.

To Tea or Not to Tea
Herbal medicines come in many forms: the dried herb that is often used to make teas, pre-made teas, capsules or tablets, balms or ointments, alcohol or glycerin extracts, and essential oils (the oil extracts of herbs). The best herbal preparation for your needs varies depending on whether you need a systemic immune system boost, have an infected skin wound, or something else altogether different. It also depends on the severity of the infection and the level of weakness of your immune system or overall strength.

In my nearly three decades of experience of using herbal medicines for healing, I have found that essential oils tend to be the most potent remedy as they are highly concentrated oil extracts of the plants from which they are derived; however, only the oil-soluble medicinal compounds are extracted into essential oils. In some cases, water soluble compounds may be needed, and in these cases typically alcohol extracts, known as tinctures, may be best. Essential oils tend to work well when used internally where appropriate, but not all essential oils are suitable for internal use. We'll explore more on the internal use of essential oils momentarily. This is just a generalization and there are many herbs and oils that break the rules.

On the flip side, using herbs in tea form, which is known as an infusion, tends to be the gentlest way to use herbal medicines. But it tends to be the least potent as well. If you're dealing with a severe infection, you may wish to use other forms of herbal medicines; however, that does not mean that you should discard herbal teas altogether, as they play important roles in helping to rebuild the body and the immune system over time. Additionally, certain herbal teas cooled and used as a mouthwash or swished in the mouth like a mouthwash can be beneficial for oral or dental infections. I've included a recipe for an herbal tea-based mouthwash later in this chapter.

Herb or Essential Oil?

The type of infection will determine both the remedy and the best means of using the remedy to achieve results. For example: In respiratory infections, diffusing key essential oils can help to get microdroplets of anti-infectious oils to both the upper and lower parts of the respiratory system, where they may begin to work quickly and effectively to deal with respiratory infections. While this particular approach may be helpful for lung infections, it is certainly not the most effective way to address blood infections, where key essential oils and herbs used internally are likely far more effective. However, diffusing essential oils can certainly play a supporting role in treating these types of infections.

Of course, it's also beneficial to consider the research, some of which I've shared for each herb, since some herbs are more effective at treating certain types of microbial infections than others. For example, thyme has shown itself to be among the most effective natural treatments for *Streptococcus mutans* (*S. mutans*). So, if you have been diagnosed with that type of infection, then you may wish to target it with this particular remedy.

In many cases, you may not know the exact name of the infection. In those cases, you may wish to peruse the herbal information below to find the ones that sound like the best fit for the types of issues or symptoms you're experiencing. You may also wish to consider the location of the infection—respiratory, skin, systemic, or another type altogether—to find remedies that have shown effectiveness in similar situations.

SAFETY FIRST

Herbal remedies have a lengthy history of safe and effective use, but that doesn't mean you should throw caution to the wind and just pop handfuls of herbal pills or ingest droppers full of tincture without regard for possible adverse effects. It's important to maximize the effectiveness of herbs by understanding some basic safety considerations. Of course, if you have any health issue or are taking any prescribed medications or over-the-counter drugs, you'll want to check first to ensure that using them alongside your health condition or mixing them with drugs is safe. Consult your physician or pharmacist.

If you have a history of alcohol abuse, are diabetic, or when using remedies with children, it is best to avoid alcohol-based preparations in favor of other forms of herbal medicines.

Internal use of essential oils is also not recommended for children or for people with ulcers or a sensitivity or allergy to the food or herb from which the oil is extracted.

Glycerites, which are liquid herbal extracts in glycerin, are often best suited for children. They are not as strong as alcohol extracts and a better option for diabetics and those with a history of alcohol abuse.

Not all remedies are suitable with children so it is best to check the product you've selected with a qualified health professional prior to use to ensure its suitability for children.

Consult your physician before using herbs or essential oils if you are pregnant or breastfeeding as few studies have been conducted on pregnant or lactating women.

As I mentioned earlier, there are additional special considerations when using the essential oil extracts of herbs, much of which is not listed on the package, so I've included some information that follows.

Special Considerations for Using Essential Oils

Some of the most powerful natural medicines are literally right below your nose yet few people ever consider them to boost their immune system or to overcome bacterial, viral, or other microbial conditions. Sadly, the beauty and personal care industries have led most people to believe that essential oils can help them relax and beautify their looks, but little more than that. While they can boost skin health, thicken hair, and help you to relax, their most impressive virtues lie in their ability to transform your health, even against serious illness.

Most people have heard of or even used essential oils, but they may not be clear what exactly essential oils are. They are the concentrated oil extracts of flowers, plants, resins, trees, and other botanical elements found in nature that have healing properties. Each oil has unique therapeutic characteristics, depending on the plant species used, the part of the plant used, the timing of its harvest, the soil and other environmental conditions in which it grew, the method of extraction, and other factors.

A particular essential oil may contain a hundred or more naturally occurring chemical constituents that produce unique and powerful effects in the body. Due to their highly concentrated nature, some experts estimate that essential oils can be forty to sixty times more potent than the herbs from which they are derived.

Even a single plant can yield different types of oils depending on the part of the plant used, such as bark, flower, fruit, leaf, or root.

Because of the hundreds of compounds, as well as the concentrated nature of essential oils and that they can be administered in a variety of ways that work quickly in the body, essential oils are powerful healers. And, when it comes to bacteria, viruses, and other microbes, they truly shine.

According to a meta-analysis published in the *International Journal of Molecular Sciences,* many different essential oils demonstrated effectiveness against cold and flu viruses (H1N1 and H9N2 specifically) including: geranium (*Pelargonium graveolens*), lemon balm (*Melissa officinalis*), tea tree (*Melaleuca alternifolia*), and thyme (*Thymus vulgaris*).[1] And, of course, that is just one example of the many studies that show how essential oils shine when they encounter infectious microbes.

Additionally, essential oils can work synergistically to boost each other's performance against bacterial and viral threats. In a study published in the medical journal *Phytotherapy Research,* scientists showed that thyme essential oil demonstrated significant antiviral activity, particularly when combined with eucalyptus and tea tree.[2]

Not all herbs have essential oil extracts. Wherever they do, or whenever essential oils are useful considerations in healing infectious conditions, I have mentioned them below under the herbs themselves.

Using Essential Oils for Optimal Healing Results

There are many ways to use essential oils, including diffusing them or mixing them with water and spraying into the air for the purpose of inhalation, applying topically, or ingesting. In my decades of experience with using essential oils therapeutically, I have found that ingestion of one or more pure oils suitable for internal use tends to yield the best effects for most bacterial, fungal, or viral infections, unless the problem area is found on the skin or respiratory system. In the case of skin infections, applying the essential oils (based on the instructions provided below) tends to yield optimal benefits, but appropriate internal use of key oils may support the immune system or help the body attack the infection from inside the body as well. In the case of respiratory infections, diffusing the oils along with using them internally as directed tends to provide a two-pronged approach that has been effective, in my experience.

Not all oils are suitable for ingestion so please follow the usage instructions that follow each herbal profile throughout this chapter. Herbs that are available in essential oil form are clearly delineated with a droplet symbol. If an herb is demarked with a droplet symbol, it is still imperative to follow the guidelines suggested since *not all essential oils are suitable for internal use.* Also, please keep in mind that most of the oils on the market are not suitable for consumption or oral use. Select oils that clearly indicate their suitability for internal use on the label. This is easily identifiable on the label, which would indicate "dose." The oil may state "not suitable for internal use," which is fairly obvious that it should definitely not be used in this manner.

Most of the herbs and oils that I've described below are potent, and in their essential oil form are even more so, so you'll want to dilute them before using. Dilution instructions follow later in this chapter. If you are inexperienced in using essential oils internally, it is best to consult with a qualified natural health expert. Internal use of essential oils is best reserved for short-term use rather than for many years, although there are some exceptions to the rule. Every product is different so it is not possible to itemize them all here. I include extensive information on essential oils and using them on my website, so please consult this resource for more information.

Make sure you select high quality, pure, undiluted essential oils. While you may end up diluting the oils yourself, most of the oils on the market are diluted in less-than-desirable oils. High quality oils cost more than the cheap varieties on the market but are worth the increased price. Many cheap varieties can also contain synthetic versions of the oils, which offer no therapeutic value and may actually be harmful. But, worse than that, many cheap oils are adulterated with solvents used during the extraction process or toxic pesticides used in the growing process of the herbs from which the oils are extracted.

After diluting the oil in carrier oil, always conduct a forty-eight-hour patch test on a small inconspicuous part of your skin to determine whether you have any sensitivity to the essential oils. Do not discontinue any prescribed medications without the guidance of your physician. Use essential oils with caution and the advice of a qualified natural health practitioner during pregnancy or in the treatment of any health condition.

Always choose high-quality oils. Most of the oils found in pharmacies, big box stores, and even many online retailers are inferior quality and not suitable for therapeutic purposes. When purchasing essential oils, like most things, you get what you pay for: higher quality oils tend to cost more. This is especially true of rare oils like melissa, or lemon balm, as it is also known. Lemon balm essential oil is often substituted with lemongrass essential oil because they have similar names and scents. While lemongrass is a beneficial oil in its own right, it has few, if any, of the antiviral properties of melissa, which is a potent antiviral oil. If you're battling a severe virus, obviously purchasing the cheap oil can have costly ramifications for your health and life.

But, melissa isn't the only type of oil that is often bastardized. Most of the cheap oils on the market are often extended with artificial or other ingredients, including many harmful ingredients like cancer-causing phthalates or petrochemical solvents. As a result, cheap oils are best avoided.

While "hot" oils like cinnamon, clove, oregano, and thyme need to be diluted with a carrier oil like fractionated coconut oil or apricot kernel oil prior to using, if you have sensitive skin you may need to dilute these and other oils as well. In the case of highly sensitive skin, you may need to avoid topical use of the hot oils, even when they are diluted. Also, keep in mind that if you are using the oil inside your mouth, you should only use products that have been approved for internal use.

Cold or Flu? How to Tell

A cold usually comes on slowly, rarely involves a fever, causes only slight aches, and chills are uncommon, while sneezing, stuffy nose, and sore throat are common. Also, a cold rarely causes headaches. Influenza comes on abruptly, usually involves fevers, aches, chills, and fatigue, while headaches are common.[3]

Cold	Flu
• comes on slowly	• comes on abruptly
• rarely involves fever or headaches	• usually involves fevers and headaches
• causes only slight aches	• usually causes aches
• uncommonly causes chills	• commonly causes chills
• commonly causes sneezing, stuffy nose, sore throat	• usually involves fatigue

INTRODUCING THE ALL-STAR REMEDIES

There are many herbs with anti-infectious properties that can give your immune system the helping hand it needs to overcome various types of infections; however, I've selected the ones that are, in my view, (1) most effective against bacterial, fungal, or viral infections; (2) excellent general anti-infectious remedies; or (3) readily available. Regarding the latter, what good does an obscure rainforest remedy do if you have to scour the Amazon jungles to find it? It's not practical at the best of times, and especially not if you're burning up with a fever from a serious condition.

I've provided dosage amounts and instructions for the herbs and essential oils below but it is best to follow the package directions for the type of product you select since there are wide variations between products. If you choose an alcohol tincture, glycerite (glycerine-extraction), or capsules, follow the dosage amount and frequency of use on the package for the product you've selected as they can vary widely.

After the name of each herb, along with its scientific name to help you ensure you're obtaining the therapeutic species, I've included a leaf symbol to represent herb 🌿, a droplet to represent essential oil 🌢, or both to represent herb and essential oil. This will help you to quickly delineate whether to use the herb in one of its forms, such as those mentioned above (tincture, glycerite, decoction, infusion, capsules, or other form) or to use as an essential oil.

Wherever the leaf symbol for an herb has been delineated, I will provide detailed information at the end of the herb profile suggesting the format that I've found to be most effective, such as tincture or decoction, and instructions for use. And, the same is true of the droplet symbol for essential oils. I will share whether the essential oil can be used internally (using a suitable product for this purpose, of course), applied topically, or diffused into the air.

Last Cautions about the Herbal Remedies

Before we embark on the journey to discover the most powerful herbal medicines that boost immunity and prevent and treat bacterial, fungal, and viral illnesses, it is important to stress again that you should always consult a physician if you are experiencing any symptoms of infection or illness. If you are currently taking other types of medications, synthetic or natural, you should research any possible reactions that the drugs may cause when combined with traditional herbal medicines, or consult an appropriate authority on the topic.

The information for these herbs, as well as all of the natural medicines in this book should not be a substitute for common sense, a skilled herbalist, or a physician. You may notice that unlike the common vernacular, I have referred to the drug reactions with herbs, not the other way around. It is nonsensical to me to suggest that the plants that have existed for thousands of years are to blame for interactions with synthetic drugs that have been manufactured for one to two hundred years maximum, and sometimes a lot fewer years than that, and are now in heavy use.

Throughout this chapter, we'll discuss the following immune-boosting and immune-supporting herbs, which include: basil, cat's claw, chamomile, cinnamon, cloves, cumin and black cumin, echinacea, elderberry, garlic, ginger, lemon balm, licorice, mandarin, olive leaf, oregano, peppermint, Siberian ginseng, star anise, tea tree, and thyme. It is not necessary, or even advisable, to take all of the herbs or essential oils listed. This information is presented to help you select the one, two, or maybe three, that may be most helpful to address specific health issues you may be facing, or to help you choose herbs or oils that might help boost your immunity to prevent infection. Of course, the herbs and oils are not panaceas that enable you to live an unhealthy lifestyle that could put you at risk of various types of infections. They should not replace common sense or other protective measures to prevent or reduce the possibility of infections. Not all of these herbs are available as essential oils. Wherever they are, I have mentioned their use; otherwise, there will be no mention of essential oils when none exist, are difficult to obtain, or are not recommended for use.

Basil ♦
(Ocicum basilicum)

You have undoubtedly heard of the herb basil and may even have one growing on a windowsill or in your garden, and indeed you may even reap the culinary rewards of fresh and dried basil, and may even have enjoyed their therapeutic benefits. However, for the purpose of supporting the immune system to conquer infectious illnesses, it warrants noting that the bulk of research that has achieved therapeutic benefits from basil have done so using the essential oil. As a result, the information contained here supports the use of the essential oil.

While research into basil essential oil's effectiveness against bacteria is in the preliminary stage, this natural remedy has shown excellent potential against various strains of bacteria. Multiple studies found that basil essential oil demonstrated antibacterial effects against the bacteria known as *E. coli*. This frequently drug-resistant bacteria are responsible for cramps, diarrhea, and vomiting linked to food poisoning, and are frequently to blame (along with various species of *Enterococcus* bacteria) for urinary tract infections (UTIs).[4]

Research reported in the journal *Molecules* found that natural volatile oils in basil even inhibited multiple *drug-resistant* strains of *E. coli* bacteria. Interestingly, the alcohol extract of the same plant was also effective against tuberculosis-causing bacteria, according to a preliminary study published in *BMC Complementary and Alternative Medicine*.[5]

Methods of Application: A typical dose is two to three drops of basil essential oil—a variety that's suitable for internal use—in empty capsules, taken three times a day for up to six weeks, then take two weeks off. I recommend using empty capsules when you're taking hot oils like cinnamon, clove, oregano, or thyme since they can burn the mucus membranes, but also with oils you don't wish to taste, and to assist the oils in getting deeper into the digestive tract.

Black Cumin/Black Seed Oil 🌿 💧
(*Nigella sativa*)

You may be familiar with the spice known as cumin since it is commonly used in Indian, Latin American, Middle Eastern, and North African cuisines. But, it's not just delicious when added to your favorite curries or taco spice mixture, cumin is also highly therapeutic. There are different types of cumin, which are totally different plants, so it is imperative that you're using the correct one. The cumin commonly used for culinary purposes is known in scientific circles as *Cuminum cyminum*,[6] while another type of cumin, known as black cumin, is primarily known for the oil extracted from it, known as *Nigella sativa*.

In a study published in the *International Journal of Molecular Sciences*, researchers found that the spice cumin demonstrated significant antibacterial and antifungal properties against a wide range of microbes, including *Bacillus subtilis, Pseudomonas fluorescens,* and *Vibrio parahaemolyticus*, as well as the fungus *Aspergillus flavus*. The spice even demonstrated antibacterial activity against the drug-resistant strain *S. aureus.*[7] You can obtain immune-supporting therapeutic benefits from the addition of cumin powder or cumin seeds to your favorite Indian curries and Mexican dishes, as well as other foods. Its savory flavor adds a delightful taste to many foods, including chili, which is one of my favorite ways to use this spice. However, if you're trying to address a serious infection, you may need to use black cumin seed oil.

Black cumin seed oil is growing in popularity due to its potency against a wide range of ailments. When it comes to the immune system and addressing disease-causing microbes, black cumin seed oil demonstrates powerful antiviral, antioxidant (it kills harmful free radicals), and anti-inflammatory properties, and also has proven its ability to dilate the bronchial passageways of the lungs. Additionally, black cumin seed oil has been found to improve breathing and reduce coughing.[8] All of these properties could explain the oil's potential against SARS-CoV-2, the virus involved in Covid-19 infections. In a study published in the *Journal of Pharmacopuncture,* researchers identified that nigellidine and alpha-hederin found in black cumin seed oil may inhibit SARS-CoV-2, the virus involved in Covid-19 infections.[9] This suggests that black cumin seed may be beneficial in the treatment of Covid-19. The oil has also demonstrated promise in pilot studies against HIV.[10]

Research published in the *Journal of Ayub Medical College* in Pakistan found that black cumin seed oil was effective in a laboratory setting at inhibiting MRSA, which is frequently serious or even deadly in humans.[11]

A growing body of scientific studies are starting to investigate and support this natural medicine, which has a lengthy history of therapeutic use. It has even shown effectiveness against multi-drug resistant bacteria.[12] In a study published in the journal *Natural Product Radiance,* researchers found that out of 144 strains of bacteria that were resistant to common drugs like amoxicillin, gatifloxicin, and tetracycline, black cumin inhibited ninety-seven of them, especially *P. aeruginosa* and *S. aureus.*[13] In other words, black cumin seed oil was effective even when these drugs were not effective against some bacteria.

In addition to the compounds mentioned earlier, three of the primarily therapeutic compounds found in black cumin seed oil include: thymoquinone (TQ), which is well-known for its antioxidant, anti-inflammatory, and anticancer effects; thymohydroquinone (THQ), which is one of the most powerful natural AChE inhibitors that are commonly used in the treatment of Alzheimer's disease, autism, glaucoma, dementia, Parkinson's disease, and schizophrenia; and thymol, which is a known antiviral and tuberculocide, meaning demonstrating the ability to inhibit the bacteria *M. tuberculosis*.[14,15]

In a study published in the *Egyptian Journal of Biochemistry and Molecular Biology,* researchers found that TQ, THQ, and thymol had 100 percent inhibition rates against thirty pathogens.[16]

Because the culinary spice cumin and black cumin seed oil are totally different, it is important not to confuse the two or use them interchangeably.

Methods of Application: Cumin essential oil can be applied diluted (see dilution guide at the end of this chapter) and applied topically to the skin for skin conditions, applied to the palms of hands or soles of feet for systemic conditions, and applied to large areas of the body that may be affected (for example, the chest for lung or respiratory conditions). It can be diffused into the air for respiratory conditions.

Black cumin seed oil is available in gel capsules. A typical therapeutic dose is three small gel caps three times daily, but follow the package directions for the product you select since gel capsule and dosage size may vary.

Cat's Claw
(*Uncaria tomentosa*)

Growing between thirty and sixty meters high, this vine can even reach seemingly unheard thicknesses of thirty centimeters, or one foot, with large claw-like appendages that help the vine to cling to the host plant. But, cat's claw's unusual name conceals the herb's potent nature. With such a name, it may be easy to cast aside any thought of it having strong antimicrobial effects, but the herb's antibacterial, antifungal, and antiviral properties have been proven effective in combating persistent infections, including those involved in bladder infections, Crohn's disease, gastritis, glandular fever (Epstein Barr syndrome), hepatitis, herpes, Lyme disease, prostatitis, and yeast infections (*Candidiasis*).[17]

A small, but growing, body of research found that cat's claw demonstrated antibacterial effects against *Enterococcus faecalis* (*E. faecalis*), a type of bacteria that has been linked to infected root canals in the mouth,[18] as well as *S. mutans* and multiple species of *Staphylococcus*.[19]

The bark lining of an Amazon rainforest plant found in Bolivia, Brazil, and Peru,[20] this tropical vine is commonly used for arthritis and other pain disorders. Cat's claw has also demonstrated significant antiviral activity, including against the herpes simplex virus[21] as well as SARS-CoV-2.[22]

Research shows that cat's claw stimulates immune system cells known as macrophages while also regulating the proliferation of other immune cells known as lymphocytes. Because of its immune-regulating properties, cat's claw is considered beneficial for immune disorders.[23]

Cat's claw contains powerful compounds, many of which have been shown to kill microbes, but it can also have side effects if not used correctly. Avoid use if you have an ulcer, gastric bleeding, or are taking blood thinning drugs, as cat's claw contains tetracyclic oxindole alkaloids (TOAs).[24] Additionally, cat's claw has been found to significantly increase the amount of antiretroviral drugs circulating in the body of those taking both products, which would require close monitoring by a physician.[25] Many commercial products have removed TOAs to reduce the potential for harmful side effects.

Consult with your physician prior to using cat's claw if you have a bleeding disorder, autoimmune disorder, kidney disease, leukemia, blood pressure disorder, or if you are awaiting surgery, as well as if you're taking any synthetic drug medicines for blood pressure, cholesterol, cancer, or blood clotting.[26]

Methods of Application: Cat's claw is available in powder, capsules, or as an alcohol extract. It is most frequently taken in capsule form. Because dosages vary widely depending on which expert is consulted, it is best to follow the package directions for the cat's claw product you select.

Chamomile
(German: *Matricaria chamomilla* or *Matricaria recutita*; Roman: *Chamaemelum nobile*)

Chamomile is a small but powerful herb. It might surprise people to learn that its most potent medicine is found in its tiny, daisy-like flowers that have white petals and yellow centers. But, don't be deceived by their delicate beauty; chamomile flowers pack an anti-infectious punch. Chamomile grows wild in parts of Europe and has been introduced to North America.

There are multiple types of chamomile, including German, Roman, Hungarian, and wild chamomile. The German type (*Matricaria chamomilla* or *Matricaria recutita*) and the Roman (*Chamaemelum nobile*) are the most common. German chamomile is an annual plant that grows as tall as three feet and can produce quite large flowers, whereas Roman chamomile is a perennial plant that grows close to the ground and has smaller flowers.

Germany's Commission E approved German chamomile as a treatment of the skin to reduce swelling and fight bacteria, as well as a tea or supplement to alleviate stomach cramps.[27] Both skin and gastrointestinal issues are frequently linked to harmful bacteria.

Chamomile demonstrates effectiveness against bacterial and fungal infections. In a study published in the *Indian Journal of Dentistry*, researchers found that German chamomile exhibits effectiveness against common dental bacteria and fungi, namely the bacterium *E. faecalis* and the fungal condition caused by *C. albicans*. The former is an antibiotic-resistant and often life-threatening condition that inhabits root-canal-treated teeth while the latter is a fungal (although more frequently referred to as a yeast) infection that can be difficult to treat.

In this study, a high-potency extract of German chamomile helped to kill both microbes.[28] This research could help explain German chamomile's reputation among herbalists for healing dental abscesses and gum inflammation.

While chamomile is not known for its antiviral effects, some preliminary research published in the *Journal of Pharmacy and Pharmacology* found that chamomile essential oil could be helpful in the treatment of drug-resistant herpes simplex-1 viruses.[29] I'm not suggesting that chamomile may not have antiviral effects, only that if it does, it is not readily known at this time.

Methods of Application: Chamomile's healing properties are derived from the flowers, which can be used fresh or dried and kept in a jar and brewed into a tea. Chamomile tea is also readily available in most health food and grocery stores. Chamomile tea can also be brewed and kept refrigerated for up to three days and used as a mouthwash to address dental infections. Simply swish the tea in your mouth for up to a few minutes. The herb is also available in extract and essential oil forms. Extracts can be taken internally to deal with infections. Chamomile essential oil can be diluted and applied topically to skin conditions. Later in this chapter, you'll learn more about diluting essential oils for topical use. Avoid using chamomile if you are allergic to ragweed. Also, the drug warfarin (Coumadin) has been found to interact with chamomile. Other blood thinners may also interact with chamomile, so it is best not to use chamomile if you are taking these drugs. Consult your physician prior to use if you are taking these or other drugs.

A chamomile infusion of one to two teaspoons of herb per cup of boiled water can be brewed for ten minutes and drunk for internal use. Alternatively, brew the infusion in the same manner, allow to cool and use as a mouthwash for dental or oral health issues. It can be covered and stored in the fridge for up to three days. The cooled infusion can also be applied as a compress using a cotton pad over skin infections or wounds. If using the tea for the latter, be sure to use sterilized vessels and jars for making the infusion and conduct proper handwashing prior to use.

Cinnamon 🌿 💧
(*Cinnamomum cassia* and *Cinnamomum zeylanicum* a.k.a. *Cinnamomum verum*)

There are many varieties of cinnamon, including true cinnamon and *Cinnamon cassia,* which is often just called cassia, or Chinese cinnamon. While the former is touted as superior to the cassia variety, when it comes to the medicinal properties of cinnamon, they are both powerful medicines in their own right. Technically, cinnamon is the bark from the tree that shares its name, which essentially makes ground cinnamon sawdust, albeit delicious sawdust. Originating from the bark of the Cinnamomum tree in China, Chinese cinnamon also grows in other parts of Asia and is the variety widely used in Chinese medicine.[30]

In a study published in the medical journal *Microbial Pathogenesis,* researchers found that cinnamon extract or essential oil have demonstrated effectiveness against both gram-positive and gram-negative bacteria, which suggests a wide range of possible antibacterial uses for cinnamon.[31]

Cinnamon essential oil is one of the most powerful natural, research-supported, anti-infectious compounds with both antibacterial and antiviral effects. In a study published in *BMC Complementary and Alternative Medicine,* cinnamon has demonstrated strong antibacterial activity against several harmful strains of bacteria, including multiple Salmonella strains (linked to food poisoning), *E. coli, S. aureus* (linked to the sometimes-deadly MRSA infections), and others.[32] The remedy exhibited excellent activity against all the selected strains tested. Another study in the same journal found that cinnamon essential oil, as well as clove essential oil, was among the most effective essential oils against some strains of bacteria.[33]

In the journal *Molecules,* researchers found that various types of cinnamon remedies were helpful in the treatment of oral and dental issues, which are frequently due to bacteria and fungi. The researchers indicated that various preparations of cinnamon that they tested showed significant antimicrobial properties against oral pathogens and the biofilms linked to them, making cinnamon potentially beneficial for the prevention and treatment of tooth cavities, periodontal disease, oral yeast infections, and other tooth and dental issues.[34]

Additional research published in the *International Journal of Molecular Sciences* found that cinnamon, as well as cloves, cumin, oregano, and thyme, demonstrated antibacterial and antifungal properties against a wide range of microbes, including drug-resistant *S. aureus*.

Cinnamon hasn't only shown effectiveness against bacteria and fungi; it has also demonstrated potency against viruses. There is good news for anyone who tends to get every flu bug going around: exciting research published in the medical journal *Microbiology Open* found that cinnamon essential oil is effective against flu viruses.[35] Other research supports cinnamon's use against the avian flu virus (H7N3). In the study published in the *Journal of Microbiology and Biotechnology* researchers found that cinnamon essential oil (*Cinnamomum cassia*) demonstrated significant antiviral activity against this virus.[36]

Methods of Application: Cinnamon powder can be added to foods on a regular basis. While I encourage this use, it isn't necessarily the best way to benefit from cinnamon's anti-infectious properties if you're dealing with an active infection or at the onset of symptoms of an infection.

Cinnamon essential oil, when using a suitable product for internal use, can be highly effective for infections, in my experience. Add a drop or two to an empty capsule and take with food three times daily. Depending on the sensitivity of your digestive tract, you may need to dilute five to ten drops of cinnamon oil in a tablespoon of extra virgin olive oil, store in a small bottle then add five drops of the blend to an empty capsule and take with food three times daily. I also find adding a drop of cinnamon essential oil to a teaspoon of honey (Manuka honey is ideal for its potent anti-infectious properties), mixing until well-combined, and consuming is ideal for the early signs of a cold or flu virus, or other types of viral or oral infections. Always heavily dilute cinnamon essential oil in a carrier oil before applying topically.

Cloves 🌿 ●
(*Eugenia caryophyllata*)

Who doesn't love the pungent and sweet smell of cloves in mulled cider, gingerbread cookies, or just about anything during the holiday season? But the holidays aren't the only time of year to show cloves a little love.

Cloves, the spice as well as the essential oil, are best known for their ability to alleviate toothaches, which is why cloves are a common ingredient in natural toothpaste and mouthwash. Additionally, cloves (which contain eugenol, known for its antipain properties) are often added to liniment and massage oils. But, cloves also have broad and potent anti-infectious properties, fighting bacteria, fungi, and viruses alike.[37]

Research found that cloves, as well as cinnamon, demonstrate antibacterial activity against *E. coli* and *K. pneumoniae* bacteria.[38]

In a study published in the journal *Mycoses*, researchers found that clove essential oil demonstrated antifungal activity against a broad range of *Candida* species.[39]

Because the mucus membranes are quite sensitive, you'll want to dilute the essential oil one to one hundred drops of a carrier oil suitable for ingestion. Also, be sure to only use clove oil that is suitable for internal use since it is absorbed through the mucus membranes. Most essential oils on the market are not pure enough for this purpose so you'll want to shop around for a suitable one.

An exciting preliminary study in the medical journal *Pharmaceutical Research* identified a compound in cloves that showed great promise as an antiviral remedy against the deadly Ebola virus, which seems to have been making a comeback.[40] Other research has shown that cloves are a broad-spectrum antiseptic, fighting bacteria and viruses alike. Clove essential oil is also one of the most powerful natural medicines against superbugs and viruses, but is rarely, if ever, mentioned in other books on immunity. It may hold promise against herpes simplex and hepatitis C viruses as well.[41] In another study published in *Phytotherapy Research*, scientists found that clove essential oil, with its dominant active component eugenol, prevented herpes simplex 1 and 2 from replicating, which they need to do for their survival.[42]

Methods of Application: While cloves and ground cloves can be used in cooking and baking, and indeed, I encourage it, if you're dealing with an infectious disease, you may need something a bit stronger than that. You can make a decoction by adding one to two teaspoons of whole cloves per cup of water in a pot, bring to a boil, then reduce and allow to simmer for forty-five minutes. Drink one to two cups daily. Dilute for topical use, as it may cause skin irritation. Add one to two drops of clove essential oil suitable for internal use to an empty capsule. Take three times daily with food. Dilute the essential oil in olive oil for internal use before adding to empty capsules if you have a sensitive gastrointestinal tract. Use with caution if you have a liver condition. Clove essential oil can be diffused in small amounts to assist with respiratory infections or issues. While clove essential oil has been found to kill many *Candida* species, suggesting its potential in addressing yeast infections, it should only be used internally, not in a vaginal douche, as it is too strong for that purpose.

Echinacea
(*Echinacea purpurea*,
Echinacea angustifolia, *Echinacea pallida*)

Even people who have never given herbal medicine much consideration have heard of echinacea—often because the mainstream media seems to love studies that claim the herb is ineffective; however, most of these studies have been poorly constructed, using ineffective varieties or doses too low to yield therapeutic results.

Echinacea is most people's go-to North American herb when they feel a virus or other infection coming on, and for good reason—because it works well, at least when quality products are used with the correct strains, in the correct potency, frequently enough to work, and for the duration needed. As with all medicines, they need to be used correctly to yield results, yet those who construct some herbal studies seem to neglect this simple fact and produce less-than-impressive outcomes as a result. But, there are many well-constructed studies on echinacea's effectiveness and a lengthy history of successful use that warrants consideration.

With a centuries-long history of use among Native Americans and the First Nations of Canada for a wide variety of ailments,[43] echinacea has become best known for use with colds, flu, and at the first sign of other infectious conditions.

David Hoffman, FNIMH, AHG, emphasizes the use of echinacea in his book *Medical Herbalism: The Science and Practice of Herbal Medicine,* indicating that it is one of the primary herbs to assist with microbial infections. He states: "It is often effective against both bacterial and viral attacks. It may be used for conditions such as boils, septicemia, and similar infections, and in conjunction with other herbs, it may be used for any infection anywhere in the body."[44]

Research published in the medical journal *Advances in Therapy* concluded that echinacea significantly reduces the risk of recurring respiratory infections, ear infections, tonsillitis, and pharyngitis.[45] This versatile herbal medicine has also been found to reduce the severity of symptoms linked to respiratory infections. In a study published in the journal *Cell Immunology,* researchers found that echinacea demonstrated potent anti-inflammatory properties that are likely responsible for these effects.[46]

According to a study published in *Virology Journal,* the herb showed antiviral activity against the common cold coronavirus as well as SARS-CoV-2.[47] Other research published in the journal *Phytomedicine* found that echinacea increased the immune system cells known as leukocytes and natural killer cells, which in turn helps to boost the overall functioning of the immune system.[48] These effects may be helpful in the prevention or treatment of a wide range of infectious conditions.

Some reports suggest that echinacea may cause allergic reactions in some people so if you suffer from allergies, be sure to do a skin patch test prior to use or to avoid it altogether if you have an allergy to echinacea. In theory, although I'm unaware of studies that support the claim, echinacea may interact with immunosuppressant therapy. While some people take echinacea as a preventative, it is more effective to use it therapeutically to treat active infections or at the first signs or symptoms of an infection.

Methods of Application: Tinctures tends to be the most effective therapeutic preparation. A treatment dose is one to four milliliters, three times daily. A decoction of the root is also effective. To make a decoction, place in a pot one to two teaspoons of dried echinacea root per one cup of water and bring to a boil. Reduce and let simmer for forty-five minutes. Strain and drink one cup, three times daily.

Elderberry
(*Sambucus nigra*)

Elderberry seemed to grow everywhere in one of the areas I lived in British Columbia, Canada. I loved going out in the fall to harvest the bounty of fruit to prepare into elderberry syrup, which is a commonly-used antiviral remedy among herbalists. Elderberry can be found growing in many parts of Canada and the United States[49] and is one of the most popular natural antiviral remedies.

Its widespread reputation among herbalists is backed by scientific research showing its effectiveness against influenza A virus[50] and other upper respiratory infections.[51,52] Other research found that elderberry extract was effective against ten strains of influenza, and it shortened the duration of influenza by three to four days, which is significant for those suffering or unable to work during that time.[53] The research on elderberry for the treatment of flu, along with many peoples' reports of benefits, suggests that it is likely among the best remedies for the treatment of flu.

In a meta-analysis published in the journal *Complementary Therapies in Medicine,* researchers found that elderberry substantially reduced upper respiratory symptoms. The scientists concluded that: "These findings present an alternative to antibiotic misuse for upper respiratory symptoms due to viral infections, and a potentially safer alternative to prescription drugs for routine cases of the common cold and influenza."[54]

There is controversy surrounding whether elderberry should be used in those with severe symptoms that might indicate a cytokine storm, largely arising out of assumptions that involve applying a drug model to herbs. In other words, drugs are typically used to increase or decrease the production of a substance in the body, or to provide the substance in lieu of the body's own production, but I am unaware of any drug that can either raise or reduce the production of a substance, depending on the body's need. Yet, many herbs can have this intelligent, balancing effect on the body. People often assume that herbal medicines function in the same way as drugs, but herbal medicines are far more complex than drugs that are made of a single or a few typically synthetic compounds.

Research published in the journal *European Cytokine Network* found that elderberry activates the immune system by increasing cytokine production.[55] Cytokines are beneficial in their ability to boost immune system functioning to overcome viruses, but potentially dangerous if production excessively increases to the point of creating cytokine storms. However, research also shows that elderberry extracts demonstrate anticytokine activity as well,[56] which suggests that they may regulate cytokine production in the body. An animal study published in the journal *Inflammopharmacology* found that elderberry diminished the inflammatory response, exerting a beneficial effect on the immune system response.[57]

Methods of Application: Fresh or dried elderberries can be boiled in water for two to three minutes, then strained to create an elderberry juice, which can be preserved through the addition of one part honey to ten parts juice and brought to a boil. Add one tablespoon to a mug of hot water and drink two to three times daily. Alternatively, prepared elderberry syrup can be purchased in most health food stores. Follow the package instructions for the product you select. I am unaware of any negative side-effects or drug interactions with elderberry.

Garlic 🌿
(*Allium sativum*)

Garlic may be considered the world's original wonder drug. Archaeological remains of garlic have been found in caves with humans from ten thousand years ago, along with a Sumerian clay tablet dating from 3000 BCE, which contains a chiseled prescription for garlic.[58] It appears that garlic was in widespread use throughout the ancient world from southern Europe to China, and was revered by Egyptians and Greeks alike for its ability to ward off disease and increase strength.[59] In more recent times, garlic was used during World War I to treat wounded soldiers' infections as well as amoebic dysentery.[60]

Garlic is still readily available around the world and has a longstanding reputation for boosting health, easing cardiovascular problems, and killing infectious microbes like bacteria, fungi, and viruses. Volumes of studies could easily be compiled confirming the antibacterial, antifungal, and antiviral properties of garlic, making the bulbous herb a great antimicrobial to incorporate into your daily diet but also to use as part of a treatment plan for infections.

Its potency seems largely due to garlic's sulfur compounds known as alliin, which are converted to allicin in the presence of certain enzymes, B vitamins, minerals, and other nutrients. According to James Duke, Ph.D., late botanist and author of many herb books including *The Green Pharmacy,* garlic contains several compounds that battle colds and flu, including allicin, which is also a broad-spectrum antibiotic.[61]

Research published in the journal *Microbes and Infection* found that not only did garlic exert potent activity against both gram-negative and gram-positive bacteria,* including drug-resistant strains of *E. coli,* it also exerted potent antifungal activity against *C. albicans,* the fungus frequently behind intestinal and vaginal yeast infections.[62]

Surprisingly little research has been done to determine garlic's

---

*This terminology refers to the broad classifications used to identify bacteria and refers to the negative or positive results of a stain test used to differentiate the microbes.

antiviral effects; however, a study in *Trends in Food Science and Technology* found that the organosulfur compounds in garlic appear to enhance the immune response and block the ability of viruses to enter the cells, which they need to do to replicate.[63]

At high doses, garlic can irritate the intestinal tract, causing nausea, diarrhea, or vomiting, as well as burning of the mouth. Anticoagulant drugs, such as blood thinners, may interfere with garlic so you should consult your physician if you are taking these drugs before consuming high amounts of garlic or garlic capsules.[64]

Methods of Application: Garlic is most potently anti-infectious in its raw state but cooked garlic is still a worthy dietary addition. The beneficial compounds in garlic can be destroyed or broken down faster when it is cooked or processed. Therefore, it is ideal to use garlic in its uncooked state, such as in salad dressings; however, you'll want to eat more than a salad dressing would yield if you're dealing with an active infection. Ideally, eat one raw clove of garlic daily. Garlic is also readily available in capsule form, usually as standardized allicin extracts. For these preparations, a therapeutic dose would be 600 to 900 milligrams of garlic, yielding 6 milligrams of allicin daily, but it is best to follow the package directions for the product you select, since potency and dosage size can vary among products.

Ginger 🌿 ●
(*Zingiber officinale*)

Ginger evokes thoughts of gingersnap cookies and gingerbread houses. Thanks to its delicious flavor, it might be easy to overlook ginger as a potent antimicrobial medicine, but it is. Used in the Ayurvedic medicine tradition of India for thousands of years, ginger's use spread throughout the world along with human migration and exploration.[65]

While most known for its effectiveness against nausea, indigestion, motion sickness, and pain, ginger is also an excellent antibacterial and antiviral remedy. A growing body of research showcases ginger's potency against these microbes, even when some antibiotic or antiviral drugs may fail,[66] which is great news as we collectively deal with superbugs with increasing drug resistance.

A study published in the journal *Molecules* found that ginger essential oil is among the best immune functioning-enhancing essential oils of those reviewed.[67]

Research published in the *Journal of Ethnopharmacology* found that fresh, but not dried, ginger was effective at inhibiting the human respiratory syncytial virus (HRSV).[68]

There are many readily available, delightful-tasting herbal teas made with ginger root that you can purchase from most health food stores. I encourage you to use the one that is straight ginger and not cut with other ingredients that have lesser value against infections. Aside from helping calm stomach distress, ginger has also shown impressive antiviral activity against the avian flu (H9N2) in animal studies.[69] The same remedy is touted by herbalists for its wide-reaching antibacterial and antiviral activity.

Ginger is believed by many people to influence bleeding times when wounded, but research conducted on those who took ginger as well as those who received a placebo did not find a difference. However, blood thinning drugs may interact with larger doses of ginger. According to the German Commission E., ginger should not be used while pregnant, although Chinese medicine suggests limited ginger use to no more than 2 grams of dried ginger during pregnancy.[70] Obviously, you'll need to use your own discretion or your physician's advice. It warrants noting that ginger essential oil is extremely concentrated and the equivalent of much higher doses of raw ginger.

Methods of Application: Ginger has so many culinary uses that it's easy to incorporate fresh ginger into your diet on a regular basis. From soups, stir-fries, and curries to baked goods, desserts, and even fermented foods, ginger works in savory and sweet dishes alike. Avoid using dried ginger wherever possible as the medicinal value is greatly diminished. Fresh ginger is always best and raw is superior to cooked. You can add a two-inch piece of fresh ginger to a juicer while making fresh fruit vegetable juices. It combines with many fruits or vegetables, including apples and carrots.

Ginger is also available in capsules as a dietary supplement. Follow package directions for the product you select. Alternatively, you can make a decoction by coarsely chopping a two- to three-inch piece of fresh ginger and adding it to a pot of water, bringing to a boil, then reducing and allowing to simmer for forty-five minutes to an hour. Add a few drops of stevia or a small amount of honey, as desired. Drink one cup hot or cold three times daily. Many health food stores also offer ginger tinctures, or alcohol extracts made with ginger root. You can take thirty drops of ginger tincture three times daily. You can also add two to three drops of ginger essential oil (choose one that's suitable for internal use) to an empty capsule and take along with food three to four times daily. Do not exceed twenty drops of essential oil internally in a day.

Lemon Balm 🌿 💧
(*Melissa officinalis*)

I grew a large batch of lemon balm, which is also sometimes referred to as melissa, from seed this year, allowing me to enjoy its delightful fragrance in my garden as well as its delicious flavor when steeped as tea. The herb's delicate flavor may lead people to underestimate its antimicrobial capacity but lemon balm has proven its antibacterial and antiviral effects in laboratory and clinical trials alike.[71]

Research in the journal *Plants* found that lemon balm essential oil contains key active ingredients known as geranial, neral, and citronellal, which demonstrated high antimicrobial activity against microorganisms it was tested against, including five disease-causing bacteria plus *C. albicans* and other fungi.[72]

Other research published in the journal *Microorganisms* found that a lemon balm-loaded hydrogel, intended for use in the mouth, successfully inhibited *C. albicans* growth in oral infections.[73] *C. albicans* infections of the mucous membranes of the mouth are commonly known as thrush.[74]

This common garden herb also demonstrates antiviral activity against the herpes simplex virus[75] likely due to its active constituents known as rosmarinic acid and other polyphenolics, which are water soluble, meaning they can be extracted by infusing the herb in water to make a tea.[76] In a study published in the journal *Natural Product Research*, scientists found that lemon balm is highly effective against the herpes simplex virus.[77] In preliminary studies lemon balm also demonstrated promise against HIV.[78] Further studies may be necessary to consider lemon balm a treatment for the disease, but given its history of safe use, along with the seriousness of HIV, it seems worth including in a treatment program.

Methods of Application: Fighting viruses never tasted so good. Even when prepared as an infusion, lemon balm's antiviral potency is evident, making it a good choice if you're prone to cold sores. Brew an infusion by pouring one cup of boiled water per two teaspoons of dried lemon balm and allowing it to steep for ten to fifteen minutes before drinking one cup, three times daily. You can also swish the cooled tea in your mouth for a few minutes as a mouthwash. A topical lotion or balm can be made or purchased and applied directly to cold sores and herpes simplex lesions. Follow package directions for lemon balm-infused hydrogel products. Alternatively, create your own by mixing one-half cup water and two tablespoons of chia seeds, allowing it to gel in the fridge for a few hours. Once thickened, add three drops of lemon balm essential oil and stir until mixed. Use one tablespoon at a time, holding it in your mouth for a few minutes before swallowing. Follow with a glass of water. Mix well before each use. Be sure the essential oil you select is suitable for internal use. For tinctures, a typical dose is 2 droppers full three times daily (2 milliliters, three times). Depending on the purity of the product you select, as well as your sensitivity to essential oils, you may be able to place one drop directly on your tongue or in your mouth.

Because lemon balm may affect the action of thyroid hormones, it is best to consult your physician if you have any thyroid conditions or if you're taking thyroid medications.

Licorice 🌿
(*Glycyrriza glabra*)

To say that licorice has a lengthy history of use is an understatement considering that the Greek author Theophrastus recommended licorice 2,300 years ago.[79] Licorice has also been used for thousands of years in Chinese medicine (which is not the same as traditional Chinese medicine, or TCM, which is a recent construct and also mistakenly used in place of the correct term, Chinese medicine). Additionally, licorice has been used for thousands of years in the Middle East. Archaeologists even found a bundle of licorice root in Tutankhamen's tomb. The ancient Indian system of medicine known as Ayurveda or Ayurvedic medicine also has a lengthy use of licorice root. While it's not clear exactly how long, Native Americans and First Nations of Canada have also used licorice for many years for the treatment of urinary tract problems, bronchial infections, coughs, and colds.[80]

Like ginseng, licorice is one of a relatively small group of herbs known as adaptogens, which have the ability to improve overall bodily health, regulate functions as needed, and give the body a boost to help it cope with physical, mental, or emotional stresses of just about any kind. In other words, adaptogens like licorice help the body adapt (like the name suggests) to just about any stress it encounters, by increasing or decreasing the body's response as necessary. In other words, licorice can increase and decrease outputs of the body to bring about balance. This makes the herb an excellent choice for the immune system since it may help regulate immune activity, and may even be beneficial to prevent deadly cytokine storms. While I am not aware of research on this topic, it seems possible given licorice's extensive use as a natural anti-inflammatory.

While the herb contains many therapeutic compounds, two antiviral compounds in particular have demonstrated antiviral activity. Known as glycyrrizin and 18-β-glycyrrhetinic acid (GA), research shows that glycyrrizin is effective against influenza, herpes simplex 1, and multiple other viruses, while GA has been found to be effective against rotavirus and HRSV.[81] It's not surprising that licorice has such a lengthy and widespread history of effective use against viruses.

Research in the cancer journal *Oncotarget* found that the compounds quercetin and isoliquiritigenin found in licorice demonstrated antiviral activity against the Epstein-Barr virus that is implicated in conditions like chronic fatigue syndrome, or myalgic encephalomyelitis, a severe condition characterized by disabling muscle weakness and wasting, balance issues, digestive problems, body and joint pain, as well as debilitating fatigue that tends to last for many months or even years.[82]

Because licorice is a potent herb, it can have harmful side-effects when misused, so it should be used with care. People with high blood pressure or kidney failure or who are taking heart medications should not use licorice. Licorice should also not be used in high quantities or for more than a few weeks at a time, without the guidance of a skilled herbal medicine practitioner or physician. Side effects are minimal, if any, if daily intake of licorice's constituent glycyrrhizin is kept below 10 milligrams. This ingredient is removed from most commercial herbal preparations of licorice root.

Methods of Application: Follow package directions for the product you select. If you are using a licorice tincture, a typical dose is 1 to 3 milliliters, three times daily, for up to three weeks. To make a decoction, put one-half to one teaspoon of dried licorice root per cup of water together into a pot. Bring to a boil then reduce heat and let simmer, covered, for forty-five minutes. Strain. Drink one cup three times daily for up to three weeks. Do not use licorice if you're taking heart or blood pressure drugs, corticosteroids, diuretics, or monoamine oxidase inhibitors.[83] Because other drugs may interact with licorice, it's best to check with your physician prior to use.

Mandarin ◊
(*Citrus reshni*)

We often think of citrus fruit for their vitamin C content and the nutrient's ability to fight off colds and flu, but research shows the essential oils derived from the peel of the fruit may also be beneficial against viruses. It may not be one of the most potent antibacterial, antifungal, or antiviral remedies, but it warrants inclusion here because of some exciting research that shows that mandarin essential oil may cut off flu viruses' ability to infect cells, thereby potentially shutting the viruses down before they can cause full blown flu.

According to a study published in *Microbial Pathogenesis,* researchers found that mandarin (*Citrus reshni*) essential oil had antiviral activity against H5N1 influenza viruses. The same study also found that some essential oils demonstrated the ability to prevent viruses from infecting cells, which is needed to ensure the virus's survival.[84]

Methods of Application: For best results, select a mandarin essential oil that is suitable for internal use. Add one to two drops, three times daily, to your water or other non-alcoholic beverages. See guidelines for using essential oils.

Olive Leaf
(*Olea europaea*)

First used medicinally in ancient Egypt where olive leaves were considered a symbol of heavenly power,[85] olive leaf has since become used around the world for the treatment of many conditions. Most people already know the health benefits of eating olive oil on a regular basis, but an increasing amount of research is showing that olive oil isn't the only therapeutic part of these trees.

The leaf of the trees are potent antioxidants, anti-inflammatory, and have long been used for their antiviral properties as well. The olive tree produces a compound known as oleuropein that is abundant in both the leaves as well as the olives. It is believed that this compound is responsible for the many health benefits of olive oil and olive leaf extract. In the early- to mid-1800s olive leaf was used to treat fevers and malaria.

A study published in the journal *Mycoses* found that olive leaf extract was effective at battling almost all bacteria and fungi it was tested against, including those found internally as well as on skin, hair, and nails, demonstrating its widespread antibacterial and antifungal properties.[86]

Olive leaf has demonstrated antimicrobial activity against a wide range of microbes, including those behind the following conditions: *Candida* infections, chronic fatigue syndrome, dental infections, ear infections, gonorrhea, hepatitis B, malaria, meningitis, pneumonia, shingles, tuberculosis, and urinary tract infections.[87]

Olive leaf has also demonstrated its antiviral properties against the viruses linked to colds, influenza, respiratory infections, and even shows promise against HIV.[88] A study published in *Biochemical and Biophysical Research Communications* found that olive leaf extract helped to inhibit infection and cellular transmission of HIV.[89]

Olive leaf tends to be safe for most uses. Some people with low blood pressure may need to exercise caution as it can reduce blood pressure and cause dizziness; however, this effect tends to be uncommon. It may irritate the stomach if the dose is too high. Dilute with water or reduce the dosage in that case.

It can cause diarrhea, acid reflux, headaches, heartburn, or stomach pain in some people. Avoid use if you're pregnant or breastfeeding, except under the guidance of a physician. Avoid use with blood pressure medications. If you are taking medications for diabetes, it is advisable to check with your physician, and if he or she agrees, to start with small amounts of olive leaf extract. Olive leaf extract may boost the effects of blood-thinning drugs like Warfarin, so you'll want to check with your physician prior to using and be monitored throughout use, if he/she agrees. Olive leaf may also interact with some chemotherapy drugs, so it is best to check with your physician prior to use.[90]

Methods of Application: Olive leaf is available in many forms in most health food stores, including extracts, dried leaf or teabags, capsules, or lotions. If you're dealing with a skin infection, select a product designed for topical use such as a lotion or balm that contains olive leaf, or add five to ten drops of a liquid olive leaf extract to your moisturizer. If you're dealing with an oral or dental infection, select either a toothpaste, mouthwash, or a liquid extract that is suitable for swishing in your mouth for a few minutes. For internal or systemic infections, the easiest way to obtain olive leaf is through an extract, either a tincture or another liquid product on the market. Use 1 to 2 milliliters of a tincture, three times daily. Olive leaf is also available in capsules ranging between 500 to 1,000 milligrams daily. Ideally divide the dose two to three times daily, up to 1,000 milligrams daily, taken with food. Olive leaf tea, while not typically as potent as other forms, is also available in most health food stores. Regardless of which type of product you select, follow the package directions for use.

Oregano
(Origanum vulgare)

Most people probably think of Greek cuisine when they think of oregano. And, it's no surprise given the herb's lengthy history of use in Greece even dating back to ancient times. Ancient Greeks believed that Aphrodite created oregano to make humans' lives happier[91]—a mission that has truly been accomplished with this herb given its capacity to wipe out infections and the nasty symptoms they often involve. For those who have not tried the herb against infections, doing so may help you to understand why ancient Greeks, and probably many modern ones as well, have found this herb contributes to their happiness.

Oregano is a powerfully antiseptic plant and well-known natural anti-infectious remedy that has been found to contain two potent compounds, carvacrol and rosmarinic acid, although there may be other still-undiscovered compounds in oregano that have antimicrobial properties. Unlike antibiotic drugs that work only on harmful bacteria, these compounds in oregano work against bacteria, viruses, fungi, and other microbes, making it a well-rounded antiseptic to keep in your natural medicine cabinet for use with any type of infection. These compounds demonstrate antibacterial, antifungal, and antiviral properties, and can be effective against strep infections, particularly strep throat[92] and bacterial pneumonia.[93]

Research published in the journal *Frontiers in Microbiology* demonstrated the effectiveness of oregano essential oil against antibiotic-resistant strep infections, which are most known for causing strep throat.[94]

Another study published in the *Journal of Virology* showed that oregano essential oil had significant antiviral activity against the flu virus (H1N1), among others.[95]

Preliminary research in the *Journal of Virology* found that carvacrol contained in oregano oil effectively inhibited HIV.[96]

Methods of Application: You can use any number of preparations of oregano, but the essential oil typically achieves the greatest results against infection. Not all oils of oregano are created equally and most have been heavily diluted prior to arriving on store shelves, so if you're dealing with a serious infection, you may wish to find a highly pure, unadulterated, undiluted oregano essential oil. Keep in mind that it is usually too strong for direct use in the mouth, and most are simply not pure enough for internal use, so be sure to choose a product that is suitable for this purpose to reap these rewards.

Also, it's important to note that many "oregano" essential oil products actually use herbal varieties that lack the medicinal or therapeutic properties of *Origanum vulgare*. Actually, some oils use marjoram, which is *Origanum majorana,* rather than oregano. Considering its scientific name looks like oregano, it's easy to understand why so many people may confuse the two. While marjoram may have some beneficial properties, it isn't a good option when you're seeking the potent antiviral or anti-infectious ability of oregano, *Origanum vulgare.*

Peppermint
(Mentha piperita)

While the herb peppermint makes most people think of candy and chewing gum, there's a lot more to this plant medicine than that. The use of peppermint as a culinary and medicinal remedy has been recorded since ancient Greece, where it was a staple of Greek cuisine and medicine. It was also used extensively in the Middle East and by Native Americans and First Nations of Canada as food and natural medicine.[97]

I wouldn't classify peppermint as one of the top herbs or essential oils for bacterial or fungal infections, but it does have antiviral properties, particularly against the herpes simplex virus. According to research by John Heinerman, a medical anthropologist and author of the book *Healing Herbs and Spices,* peppermint is a potent remedy against viruses, including the herpes simplex virus that causes cold sores. Heinerman found that two cups of hot peppermint tea daily were effective to alleviate symptoms and reduce the duration of herpes outbreaks. While the herpes virus is always present in the body after a person has contact with it, it can remain dormant, so periodic peppermint tea drinking can help reduce future chances of outbreaks.[98]

Peppermint is also a traditional treatment for colds, influenza, and fevers linked to them or other conditions. While a fever can be beneficial to engage the body's immune system to fight infectious microbes, it can become excessive and needs attention to prevent damage to the body.

Methods of Application: One of the best ways to reap the anti-infectious and fever-reducing benefits of peppermint is to use one to two drops of an essential oil suitable for internal use directly on your tongue, a few times daily. Over the years, I have had numerous people report that use of peppermint tea or peppermint essential oil drops rapidly reduced their fever, even when other methods weren't working. It may require repeated doses (usually two or three) to achieve this outcome.

Alternatively, you can put two to three drops of peppermint in an empty capsule, three times daily. Of course, make sure it is a pure, therapeutic-grade essential oil suitable for this use. To make an infusion of dried peppermint leaves, add one teaspoon of leaves per cup of boiled water and allow to steep for ten to fifteen minutes. Drink one to three cups a day to assist with fevers or for peppermint's antiviral properties. While there are reports that peppermint shouldn't be used with digestive conditions, peppermint has been used for many years as a digestive aid and I have personally only ever experienced digestive benefits from using peppermint. Ultimately, make the choice that's best for you in this regard. You can also obtain peppermint gel capsules or capsules that may be beneficial for their antiviral and fever-reducing properties. Follow package instructions for the product you select. I am unaware of any drug interactions or complications linked to peppermint.

6 Research-Supported Essential Oils for Cold Sores

Most people have experienced a cold sore at some point in their life thanks to the herpes virus. Let's face it: that cold sore can leave you feeling less-than-thrilled about making a public appearance and cause discomfort you'd rather avoid. Fortunately, certain essential oils can not only reduce the symptoms, but also help to combat the underlying virus. Here are some of the best research-supported options:

Chamomile: As you learned earlier, chamomile essential oil has been found to be effective against the herpes virus, the virus behind cold sores. A study published in the *Journal of Pharmacy and Pharmacology* found that chamomile essential oil demonstrated effectiveness even when the drug acyclovir did not.[99]

Cloves: Who doesn't love cloves in spice cake? But there's more to this delicious spice than just flavor. In a study published in the *Journal of Dentistry* researchers found that clove essential oil was as effective as the drug benzocaine for alleviating topical pain, making it an excellent choice for the pain of cold sores.[100]

Lemon balm: Known also as melissa, Lemon balm essential oil is a potent antiviral natural medicine. In a study published in the medical journal *Phytotherapy Research*, lemon balm essential oil even demonstrated effectiveness against herpes virus strains that did not respond to the common drug acyclovir.[101] Many of the products sold under the name lemon balm or melissa are actually lemongrass, which smells almost identical but has significantly less antiviral activity than lemon balm. So, buyer beware: Melissa/lemon balm essential oil is normally expensive to extract, making the products expensive too. If you have found a cheap oil, there is a good chance it is not lemon balm at all and is unlikely to yield the antiviral outcome for which you purchased it. Sadly, other than independent laboratory tests there is no good way of knowing for sure.

Oregano: In a study published in the journal *Food Chemistry*, researchers found that almost everyone's favorite antimicrobial oil—oregano—demonstrated mild antiviral activity against the herpes virus.[102] That might not sound too promising, but when you consider that the herpes virus is quickly becoming resistant to the drug options, mild antiviral activity is better than none at all. But, you may be surprised to learn that some companies substitute marjoram essential oil since its scientific name is similar to oregano and can easily dupe even the most alert consumers. Check out the section on oregano to learn more.

Peppermint: When it comes to controlling the viruses behind cold sores, melissa and peppermint are the oils of choice. In a study published in the journal *Phytomedicine,* researchers found that peppermint exhibited extremely high potency against the herpes virus, even against strains that do not respond to the drug acyclovir.[103]

Tea Tree: Also known as melaleuca essential oil, tea tree oil demonstrated mild antiviral activity against the herpes virus in a study published in the journal *Letters in Applied Microbiology*. I mention it here because it is the go-to oil for many people who suffer from cold sores, but it may not be the best option. Having said that, because it has slight activity against herpes viruses it is better than nothing if it is the only oil you have at your disposal.[104]

Siberian Ginseng
(*Eleutherococcus senticosus*)

One of a relatively small group of herbs known as "adaptogens," Siberian ginseng like its other adaptogenic counterparts helps the body to adapt by having a non-specific action. In other words, adaptogens act intelligently in the body, increasing or decreasing certain compounds as necessary. This term is often misused by the public and bloggers, which is not surprising given the fact that there's nothing that can do this (that I'm aware of) in synthetic drug medicine.

While Siberian ginseng is not a primary herb that I would select for treating infection, it is an excellent adjunct herb to support the body in recovery and to help prevent the immune system from overworking.

Cardiac (hypo- and hyper-tensive) and hypoglycemic drugs may interact with Siberian ginseng. In some studies, the herbal medicine seemed to increase the efficacy of the antibiotic drugs monomycin and kanamycin.[105] If you're taking these drugs or other antibiotics, be sure to consult your physician since he or she may need to adjust your dosage.

Methods of Application: According to clinical research, fifty to one hundred drops is an effective dose, taken three times daily. The recommended course of treatment is six weeks, followed by a two-week break.[106]

Star Anise
(Illicium verum)

The beautiful star-shaped spice known as star anise, which has a heavenly scent similar to licorice, is rarely used in Western cooking or even natural medicine in North America, but has a lengthy history of use in Chinese medicine and in Chinese cooking. Star anise warrants consideration for further use in the West based on its antifungal and antiviral properties that are increasingly being the topic of exploration in scientific studies. Pharmaceutical giants are well aware of the usefulness of this herbal medicine as they originally extracted shikimic acid from star anise prior to synthesizing it in laboratories to make the antiviral drug Tamiflu.[107]

There are two types of star anise: Chinese and Japanese, which look identical, so it is important to ensure you have the correct type for maximum effectiveness. Chinese star anise tea has a lengthy history of use and was used with some degree of effectiveness during the swine flu outbreak among Malaysians in 2009, although this statement is largely anecdotal in nature since it's unclear whether researchers followed up on the testimonies. Chinese star anise is *Illicium verum* while Japanese star anise is *Illicium anisatum*. Shikimic acid was originally isolated from Chinese star anise and currently the research has been conducted on this variety as well, making it the option of choice.[108]

Methods of Application: To make a tea, place a few star anise florets per cup of water in a pot and bring to a boil. Reduce heat, cover, and let simmer for forty-five minutes before drinking two to three cups daily as a treatment for viral conditions. There is little long-term safety data so it's best to use for acute conditions and then discontinue after a few weeks. Avoid use with infants and small children.

You can also diffuse star anise essential oil (make sure it is star anise, and not just anise or anise oil since they are not the correct products to use for therapeutic purposes). Follow instructions for diffusing essential oils.

Tea Tree ◆
(*Melaleuca alternifolia*)

Tea tree evokes strong memories of driving through the countryside in Australia years ago. Suddenly, the pungent aroma of tea tree filled the air as we neared a tea tree plantation. The scent was so strong that it could be smelled a mile before the plantation was even visible.

Tea tree's powerful aromatic compounds not only give the trees their intense smell, they may also play a role in the oil's potency against harmful microbes. While other parts of the tea tree may be used by the indigenous people of Australia, it is largely used for its essential oil among people around the world. Tea tree essential oil, which is often just called tea tree oil, has antibacterial, antifungal, and antiviral properties, making it a necessity for every natural home medicine kit or purse. Additionally, tea tree oil has the proven ability to break down biofilms, further assisting the body in overcoming bacterial infections.

Biofilms are a thin, potentially health-damaging layer of microorganisms that secrete substances to help ensure their survival in or on the body. Bacterial superbugs often thrive because they've learned to create these sticky layers of microorganisms, and their secretions make it difficult for the immune system to identify and overcome them. Research published in the journal *ScienceDirect* found that tea tree oil is effective against MRSA and the biofilms these bacteria create.

Other research in the *Journal of Antimicrobial Chemotherapy* found that tea tree oil contains two natural compounds known as alpha terpineol and linalool, which they attribute to its effectiveness against MRSA.[109]

As if that wasn't enough reason to love this remedy, research in the medical journal *Molecules* has also found that tea tree oil prevents influenza viruses from entering the cells, which could reduce the likelihood of getting sick.[110]

Methods of Application: Depending on the type of infection, tea tree oil can be applied to the skin or diffused in the air. While other forms of tea tree may be available or used for traditional purposes, the essential oil is the most readily available and seemingly most effective preparation to support the immune system in dealing with infectious diseases.

Thyme 🌿 💧
(*Thymus vulgaris*)

While thyme is primarily known for its delicious addition to savory meat, poultry, vegetable, and legume dishes, it is also one of the best anti-infectious herbs with a broad spectrum of applications against microbes.

In a review of thyme, oregano, and basil essential oils published in the *Journal of Microbiology and Biotechnology,* researchers found that all three were effective against a wide variety of bacterial stains. In their assessment of the essential oils' effects on *E. coli,* the researchers found that both thyme and oregano were the most effective.[111] Research published in the scientific journal *Molecules* found that thyme, as well as oregano, demonstrated the greatest effectiveness against a range of bacteria as well as fungi known as yeasts that are responsible for urinary tract infections, including the bacteria *E. coli* and as well as the fungi *C. albicans* and *Candida famata* (*C. famata*).[112]

Additional research published in the *BMC Complementary and Alternative Medicine* explored the effectiveness of a range of essential oils against various bacteria and found that thyme essential oil was the most effective against the bacteria *S. mutans*.[113]

Thyme has also been found to be effective against Aspergillus spores, which is a common type of mold that is linked to the respiratory condition known as aspergillosis, as well as against *Candida*, which is the culprit behind many intestinal, oral, or vaginal infections. In a study published in the *Brazilian Journal of Microbiology*, researchers found that not only was thyme effective at inhibiting fungal growth, it also increased the ability of the drug fluconazole to kill the disease-causing fungi.[114] A study published in the journal *BMC Complementary and Alternative Medicine* found that thyme was even effective against drug-resistant strains of *Candida*.[115]

Research published in the journal *Phytotherapy Research* found that thyme essential oil demonstrated antiviral properties. In this study, researchers assessed the merits of thyme essential oil, along with eucalyptus and tea tree essential oils, to prevent infection, and found that this combination prevented infectivity by more than 96 percent.[116] Using these oils throughout periods of time when infection risk is high, such as during the winter or when there are known infections running through communities, may significantly reduce the risk of infection.

James Duke, Ph.D., author of *The Green Pharmacy*, recommends using one teaspoon of dried thyme per cup of boiled water, steeping the herb for about ten to fifteen minutes to make thyme tea. Drink three cups daily for maximum effectiveness.[117]

Methods of Application: Diffuse thyme essential oil in the air on a regular basis throughout times of greater risk of infection, such as during the winter, to help prevent risk of viral infection. Thyme essential oil can be diluted and applied to the chest to help prevent respiratory infections. Two to three drops of pure therapeutic grade thyme essential oil can be added to empty capsules and taken three times daily to help prevent or address infections. Be sure that the product you select is suitable for internal use and preferably one with third-party laboratory verification attesting to its purity. Use thyme or thyme essential oil with caution during pregnancy. Dilute heavily for topical or for oral use if you have gastrointestinal issues. Thyme is also available in a tincture form. Use approximately 2 to 4 milliliters three times daily. Follow directions for the product you select.

I'm unaware of any drug interactions with thyme, but if you're taking any medications or have any health issues, it's best to consult with your physician prior to use.

METHODS OF HERBAL AND ESSENTIAL OIL USE FOR BEST RESULTS

Herbal Remedy	Method of Use*
Basil	Essential Oil
Cat's Claw	Capsule, Tea, Tincture
Chamomile	Tea, Tincture
Cinnamon	Capsule, Dried Herb (baking, cooking), Tea
Clove	Tea, Essential Oil
Cumin (Black Cumin)	Oil
Echinacea	Capsule, Tea, Tincture
Elderberry	Capsule, Juice, Syrup, Tea, Tincture
Garlic	Capsule, Fresh Herb (baking, cooking), Tincture
Ginger	Fresh Herb, Juice, Tea, Tincture
Lemon balm	Capsule, Dried Herb (baking, cooking), Tea, Tincture
Licorice	Capsule, Dried Herb (baking, cooking), Tea, Tincture
Mandarin	Essential Oil
Olive Leaf	Dried Herb, Tea, Extract, Tincture
Oregano	Capsule, Dried Herb (baking, cooking), Tea, Tincture
Peppermint	Essential Oil, Tea, Tincture

*Because drug-herb interactions and medical contraindications are common, it is best to follow package instructions for the product you select and consult your physician regarding any possible conditions you may have and drugs you may be taking. Follow the guidelines for internal use of essential oils as most oils are not suitable for this purpose.

METHODS OF HERBAL AND ESSENTIAL OIL USE FOR BEST RESULTS (*continued*)

Herbal Remedy	Method of Use*
Siberian Ginseng	Capsule, Dried Herb, Tea, Tincture
Star Anise	Essential Oil
Tea Tree	Essential Oil
Thyme	Dried Herb, Essential Oil

*Because drug-herb interactions and medical contraindications are common, it is best to follow package instructions for the product you select and consult your physician regarding any possible conditions you may have and drugs you may be taking. Follow the guidelines for internal use of essential oils as most oils are not suitable for this purpose.

HOW TO USE ESSENTIAL OILS

Because essential oils are highly concentrated, they are potent natural medicines that should be carefully used. By some estimates, they are between forty and sixty times stronger than the herbs from which they are derived, and that means there are some unique considerations for their safe use. A little goes a long way, so you'll only need a drop or a few drops at a time, depending on the oil and the intended use.

It is best to use essential oils as directed on the product label. As an example, if it says "for external use only" don't use it internally. In addition to the safety measures presented previously and with each remedy throughout this book, here are some additional considerations:

- Conduct a skin patch test before using any essential oil by applying a small amount of a diluted essential oil on the inside of your arm and waiting forty-eight hours to determine whether you might have a sensitivity to the oil that presents itself in the form of a rash or hives. If you do, avoid using that oil either topically or internally as you may have a sensitivity or allergy to it. If you don't have a reaction, feel free to use the remedy as directed on the package or in this book. Do not use any product in a way that it was not intended as stated on the label.
- Some oils, known in the industry as "hot oils" always need to be diluted before use. These oils include: cinnamon, clove, oregano, thyme, among

others. Dilute them by using a carrier oil like fractionated coconut oil (a liquid version of coconut oil) or apricot kernel oil. A carrier oil is a gentle oil used to dilute essential oils to make them suitable for topical use. If you wish to use suitable hot oils for internal use after conducting a skin test, dilute in some olive oil first. Hot oils are typically diluted in a ratio of one drop to one teaspoon of carrier oil.

- If you're planning to use essential oils internally, choose only products whose labels clearly indicate their suitability for internal use, otherwise avoid this use altogether.
- Avoid applying essential oils directly to the delicate membranes of the eyes and mouth, or genital areas.
- When used topically, some oils can cause photosensitivity—that means they can make your skin more sensitive to the sun. These oils typically include citrus and bergamot oils, most of which are great for a wide variety of reasons, but may not make my top immune-boosting picks; but if you're using them, please be aware of their tendency to make the skin more sensitive to sunlight. Avoid using them on your skin within several hours of direct sun exposure.

There are three main ways to use essential oils: aromatically (inhaling their lovely scents), topically (applying them on your skin), or internally (either placing them on your tongue or consuming them in food, beverages, or empty capsules). Not all oils are suitable for all types of uses, in fact most are not suitable for internal use, so be sure to read the labels on the products you select.

Aromatic Uses

When you smell essential oils, you're actually breathing in potent oil-based plant extracts of essential oils wafting in the air, sending signals directly from the cells in the nose to the brain. The brain then sends messages back to the body in response to the signals it received. These signals vary, depending on the scent (or scents) and its chemical constituents, and produce different effects—they can reduce inflammation, relax the nervous system, boost mood, reduce pain, target harmful microbes, or perform other actions. Inhaling essential oils is a quick way to allow their molecules to access the brain—usually in a minute or less. While this method is a powerful way to address infections in the sinuses and lungs, as well as to help relax the nervous system, alleviate stress, boost mood, and improve sleep, it is less effective in alleviating skin infections than topical or internal use. That doesn't mean it isn't beneficial for use in skin infections, but it plays more of a supporting role than the lead role.

The most common way to use essential oils aromatically is to place one to five drops in an aromatherapy diffuser. I don't recommend using oil burners as the heat can damage the chemical makeup of the oils, reducing their effectiveness and even causing them to smoke, contributing to respiratory irritation or inflammation, as well as to other health problems.

Topical Uses

Applying essential oils on the skin allows them not only to address localized or widespread pain conditions but also to quickly penetrate the skin and gain access to the bloodstream. Here are some of the ways in which you can use essential oils topically:

- Add a few drops of the selected essential oil or oils to a teaspoon of carrier oil like fractionated coconut oil. The level of dilution will depend on the oil and the skin sensitivity of the person on whom it will be applied. Apply the diluted oils over the affected areas (i.e., massage the oil onto the chest area to assist with respiratory infections). Avoid the skin around the eyes (unless you're using a product specifically formulated for this purpose), the eyes themselves, the inner ears, and broken or damaged skin. If you're using the oils over infected areas of the skin, you'll need to take extra precautions regarding hygiene to prevent further infecting the area.
- Add a few drops of essential oils to a teaspoon of carrier oil and add to a hot bath. Soak for ten to twenty minutes to help alleviate fevers, muscle pain linked to infections, or to help with skin or respiratory

issues. Some oils that have strong heating or cooling effects, such as birch, clove, ginger, oregano, peppermint, thyme, and wintergreen, are not suitable for this purpose as they can irritate sensitive areas of the body.

- Add a couple of drops to an old, but clean, facecloth that has been soaked in either hot or cold water and wrung out. Use as a hot or cold compress over painful areas. Cover the compress with a dry cloth to help retain its temperature. Do not use hot compresses on inflamed areas. I recommend using an older facecloth since the oils may stain the fabric.

Internal Uses

Over two decades ago, long before essential oils were popular in the natural health community, I learned about a practice of using high grade essential oils internally to effect rapid and significant healing results. At first, I was hesitant to incorporate it into my practice because I knew that, in North America at least, the approach was non-traditional and even frowned upon by a certain offshoot of classically trained aromatherapists. I set to work experimenting on myself since I wanted to be sure of their effects prior to using them in my practice. To my amazement, and contrary to what I had been taught, I had impressive results. I overcame health challenges that had eluded me. I recovered from infectious conditions faster than ever before, and I began to feel better than I had in a long time.

Fortunately, the company's owners and managers whose essential oils I was using at that time had extensive experience in the practice and had even created excellent guidebooks to help me navigate this new realm safely. They also produced products intended for internal use that were formulated for specific conditions, making it easy to ensure their safe use.

When I felt confident enough in this novel approach to using essential oils, I began incorporating them into my practice, with astounding results. I found people achieved greater results than with many of the other types of natural, and sometimes drug, options. Whether they battled infectious skin conditions, resistant yeast infections, tooth or gum infections, or some other health issue, most resolved faster and with greater effectiveness than using other remedies.

And, even all these years later, I periodically still get someone from a traditional school of aromatherapy writing some inflammatory language in an email, on a review, or as a comment on my blogs, telling me that using essential oils in this way is ill-advised. To which I always respond: "Have you tried using pure, therapeutic-grade essential oils suitable for ingestion or oral use in this manner?" Of course, the answer is always, "no." While I am well aware that there are conservative schools of thought on this process, I also know that a longstanding tradition of their safe oral use continues, and that I have had the best results with this practice, and found oils used in this way to be more effective than most other natural medicines.

Of course, not all essential oils are safe to be used in this manner. The oils from some plants are simply unsuitable for internal use of any kind. Caution needs to be exercised when using essential oils internally, but when some safety guidelines are followed, there are few, if any safety concerns, and certainly far fewer than for the average pharmaceutical drug, yet few people have concerns about taking drugs that have an enormous list of side effects, even from their "correct" use.

Considering the effectiveness that I have witnessed and their safety when following my suggestions below, how could I not share this information in good conscience knowing that they have worked when all else has failed? I have seen them save lives, or at least prolong life until medical interventions can be used. I have seen them work against serious, life-threatening infections, even when many antibiotics have failed. I would be remiss if I didn't share these remedies and how to use them at a time in our history when we're facing resistant bacterial and viral infections and many superbugs.

Many aromatherapy practitioners lack training in the use of essential oils beyond aromatherapy—the art and science of using essential oils aromatically—and therefore lack an adequate understanding of essential oils as natural medicines. This lack of knowledge often means that they discourage people from using one of the most effective methods of countering infectious diseases, including bacterial, fungal, and viral infections, through the oral use of suitable essential oils. I used these methods in my practice for many years to help women and men put an end to their suffering with exceptional results, even when little else worked. While some oils are not suitable for this purpose and there are safety precautions to consider, keep in mind that most people naturally ingest some amount of essential oil in the plant-based foods and herbs they eat every day.

When done correctly, ingesting essential oils can be the most effective way to experience their benefits. Once you ingest a suitable essential oil, the oil compounds enter the bloodstream through the gastrointestinal tract, where they are transported to all the tissues and organs, providing assistance to the immune system in its effort to overcome infectious diseases.

As with anything that is consumed, it is imperative to use appropriate doses to avoid toxicity—the point at which even the healthiest of substances becomes unhealthy or harmful. If you're considering using essential oils internally, you'll need to determine whether the oils are suitable for internal use and, if so, how much to use and in which format—whether it is a capsule or a drop of oil taken directly or under the tongue, or another method.

Finding the highest-quality essential oils is even more important when you'll be using them internally. If the products you've selected are appropriate for internal use, they will have "for internal use," "dosage amount," or something similar on the labels. If the labels do not indicate anything like that, avoid using the products internally, since they are likely to have contaminants that are too toxic for such use.

Once you've selected the purest oils, you'll still want to check to be sure the individual oil is suitable for internal use. For example, some brands of high-quality peppermint are fine for internal use, but star anise should not be used this way. Of course, it is not the only oil that should not be used internally. Following are some ways to use essential oils internally:

- Place a few drops of suitable, pure essential oils in empty capsules, which are available in most health food stores. Take the capsules with a glass of water, along with some food. Some oils, like cinnamon, clove, oregano, and thyme, need to be diluted with a little fractionated coconut or olive oil before ingesting. Follow the package label for the specific oil you've selected.
- You can also purchase preformed essential oil supplements to target infections, including blends that have anti-infectious properties, like OnGuard, or peppermint gel capsules. I cannot state this point frequently enough: it is imperative to exclusively choose products that are high quality.
- Regardless of why you're using essential oils internally, start slowly, using only a drop or two at a time, a few times daily. Do not exceed twenty drops within a twenty-four-hour period.

More Ways to Use Essential Oils for Immune Support

Essential oils can be diffused into the air using aromatherapy diffusers that are available at most health food stores or through companies that sell essential oils. They can also be made into ointments, massage oil blends, and other topical remedies to address the symptoms linked with bacterial, fungal, or viral infections, as well as to boost immunity against these microbes. Some, but not all, oils can even be used internally, as long as you follow some important safety guidelines. Using essential oils on a regular basis through inhalation on a cloth, diffusing in the air, or diluting and applying to your skin may not just help you after you get a cold or flu, doing so may help to prevent you from getting sick in the first place.

RECIPES FOR RELIEF

Knowing the best anti-infectious essential oils is great, but how can you use them for symptom relief when you're suffering under the weight of a nasty flu or something much worse? Try out these essential recipes the next time you become the unwitting host to an unwanted microbe.

Note: Be sure to conduct a seventy-two-hour skin patch test to determine possible sensitivities or allergies before using the oils.

◊ Honey-Thyme Cough Alleviator ◊

Combine two of the best natural cough medicines and you get this sure-fire cough reliever. While unpasteurized honey is sooth- ing to the throat in its own right, choose manuka honey to further increase the antiviral effects of this remedy. Be sure the thyme essential oil you select is suitable for internal use as not all oils are suitable for this purpose.

⅓ cup (80 mL) unpasteurized honey or manuka honey
6 drops thyme essential oil

In a small bowl, stir honey and thyme essential oils until well combined. Store in small jar and stir before use to incorporate essential oils. Use 1/2 to 1 tsp (2 to 5 mL), as needed, to soothe a sore throat or ease a cough.

◊ Peppermint Headache Relief Rollerball ◊

If you have a pressure headache that is often associated with colds, flu, and other viral infections, you'll want to have this remedy on hand. Glass rollerballs are available in most natural health stores.

10-mL glass rollerball bottle
½ teaspoon + 10 drops peppermint essential oil
7 mL (1½ teaspoons) fractionated coconut or apricot kernel oil

Remove the lid and rollerball from the glass bottle. Add essential oils. Top up with coconut or apricot kernel oil. Replace rollerball top and lid and gently roll between your hands to combine ingredients.

For headache relief, roll over the scalp up to a few times daily. Use as needed over temples, forehead, and back of the neck where the skull and neck meet. Avoid use near the eyes.

◊ Tummy Tamer Rollerball ◊

GI infections and even systemic viruses can make everything feel "off," including digestion. If you're experiencing nausea, stomach aches, indigestion, or other gastrointestinal symptoms, you'll want to keep this remedy handy.

10 mL glass rollerball bottle
15 drops ginger essential oil
10 drops peppermint essential oil
10 drops fennel or anise essential oil
Fractionated coconut or apricot kernel oil

Remove the lid and rollerball from the glass bottle. Add essential oils. Top up with approximately 1½ teaspoons (7 mL) coconut or apricot kernel oil. Replace rollerball top and lid and gently roll between your hands to combine ingredients.

For abdominal relief, roll over the abdominal area, as needed, up to a few times daily.

◊ Eucalyptus and Tea Tree Chest Rub ◊

Most of us are familiar with the vaporizing scent of eucalyptus. Many of our parents rubbed it on our chests when we had a head cold or flu. Here's a natural option free of the petrochemicals typically found in these types of ointments. It helps clear the sinuses and open the airways.

Makes approximately ⅔ cup (160 mL).

2 tablespoons (30 mL) grated beeswax (using cheese grater or
    potato peeler)

½ cup (125 mL) fractionated coconut or extra-virgin olive oil

50 drops (½ teaspoon) eucalyptus essential oil

25 drops (¼ teaspoon) tea tree essential oil

1 5-oz. ointment jar or tin

In a small pot, over low heat, heat beeswax and fractionated
coconut or olive oil, stirring gently but constantly, until beeswax
is melted. Immediately remove from stove and add eucalyptus
and tea tree essential oils; stir until combined. Immediately pour
mixture into clean glass jars or tins, leaving it undisturbed and
uncovered until completely cooled. Cover and label.

The ointment lasts about one year. Rub on your chest as needed.

Essential Oils that Support the Treatment of Lyme Disease

Most people assume that antibiotic drugs are our most potent
weapon against disease but, when it comes to Lyme disease, a recent
study suggests otherwise. Scientists at the Department of Molecular
Microbiology and Immunology at the Johns Hopkins Bloomberg
School of Public Health in Baltimore, Maryland, found that certain
essential oils were more powerful in the treatment of the bacteria
that cause Lyme disease—*Borrelia burgdorferi* (*B. burgdorferi*)—than
the standard antibiotic treatment. The study found that ten of the
thirty-five essential oils tested in laboratory dishes demonstrated
"strong activity" against the latent, "persister" forms of Lyme disease. The oils include garlic, myrrh, thyme, cinnamon, allspice, cumin,
eucalyptus, litsea, lemongrass, and spiked ginger lily.[118]

"Persister" forms of Lyme disease are considered to be those in
the 10- to 20-percent range that do not respond to the standard

antibiotic treatment, and which can be particularly challenging to those dealing with the condition.

Even in concentrations of one part to one thousand, which is considered a low dose, several of the essential oils completely destroyed the bacteria behind the disease in only seven days. What's more: there was no bacterial regrowth with these essential oils after twenty-one days.

Led by Ying Zhang, M.D., Ph.D., a professor at the school and head of the study said in an interview with Medical News Today, "We found that these essential oils were even better at killing the 'persister' forms of Lyme bacteria than standard Lyme antibiotics."[119]

That's great news for the many people diagnosed with this debilitating disease that medical experts believe to be caused by the bacterial infection B. burgdorferi linked to tick bites. Some of the symptoms of Lyme disease include: rashes (including the signature rash that looks like a bulls-eye), fatigue, achy or swollen joints, headaches, dizziness, fever, night sweats, sleep disturbances, cognitive decline, sensitivity to light, coordination problems, heart inflammation, anxiety, depression, chest pain, jaw pain, and unexplained pain.[120]

An earlier study, published in Frontiers in Medicine, confirmed the efficacy of essential oils against Lyme disease. In that study, researchers found oils of oregano, clove, and cinnamon were highly effective against the infection. The results, which "completely eradicated all viable (bacterial) cells" were believed to be as a result of such naturally occurring compounds as carvacrol in oregano.[121] Carvacrol has been shown in many studies to be anti-infectious against bacteria.

Does that mean you should throw away the antibiotic prescription your doctor gave you? Of course not. Antibiotics that have not shown resistance to the bacteria involved in Lyme disease can be important in treating this condition. But, it's also worth considering essential oils in your treatment of this often-debilitating condition.

4

Probiotics and Fermented Foods

Pro-Powered Microorganisms

You may have heard the adage that great health begins in the gut. When it comes to building a powerful immune system, that couldn't be truer.

Your gut actually houses approximately 70 percent of your immune system.[1] Located within your gut, there are an enormous number of immune system cells that combine to make gut-associated lymphoid tissue (GALT). Some of these immune cells include: B-cells, T-cells, and macrophages, among others.[2]

This first-line defense system works remarkably well until it becomes damaged or impaired in some way. Perhaps we overuse or misuse antibiotics or other medications, drink insufficient amounts of water, eat excess sugar, eat prepared or processed foods replete with chemical preservatives and colors, eat excessive amounts of meat including processed types, live a sedentary life, or participate in some other lifestyle factors that can damage the gut tissue and throw off its delicate microbial balance. But, it's not all doom and gloom.

The great news is that our bodies are miraculous in their ability to heal when we give them what they need to do so. One of the best things we can do for a healthy gut and immune system is help to restore microbial balance through the use of natural food and beverage choices, exercise, and getting more probiotics in our diet. Probiotics are "live microorganisms that, when administered in adequate amounts, confer a health benefit on the host."[3] They are readily available in fermented foods like sauerkraut, kimchi, miso, yogurt, kombucha, and other foods, provided they have not been pasteurized and, of course, are also available in supplement form.

In this chapter, we'll explore some of the best ways to get more probiotics and prebiotics into your diet to help restore gut health and immune health. It's interesting to note that a growing body of research is also finding that specific probiotics may be useful to target particular harmful bacteria or viruses, a revolutionary new approach to super-immunity that I discuss in my upcoming book *Super-Powered Immunity Starts in the Gut*.

Before we delve deeper into the microscopic world of probiotics and prebiotics, let's first discuss your microbiome and why it is important to maintaining strong health.

WHAT IS A MICROBIOME?

Our bodies contain over one trillion microscopic bacteria from approximately one thousand species,[4] which are collectively known as our microbiome. Before you gasp with disgust, it's important to know that these microbes not only keep you healthy, they ensure your survival. And, within our overall microbiome, we have collections of microorganisms that are unique to our face, right hand, intestines, or other part of our body, each of which is a smaller microbiome within the larger one. Similar to a fingerprint, our microbiome is unique to us. No one else has exactly the same microbiome as you. And, even your left and right hands have unique microbiomes.

And, as scientist Philip C. Calder stated in his study published in *BMJ Nutrition, Prevention & Health,* "The gut microbiota plays a role in educating and regulating the immune system."[5] This seemingly simple, but profound, statement might give you some insight into the importance of ensuring a healthy gut replete with beneficial bacteria, since they will help to train and regulate your immune system.

INTRODUCING THE PROS—PROBIOTICS, THAT IS

If you look on the label of a bottle of probiotics or the ingredients in a package of yogurt, one of the first things you'll see are the various probiotics in the genus *Lactobacillus,* which are usually listed on food packaging as *L.,* followed by the various strains, such as *L. acidophilus, L. bulgaricus,* and others. These probiotics tend to have an affinity for the small intestines. *Lactobacilli* convert various types of sugars to lactic acid. They are commonly found in many fermented foods like yogurt, fermented vegetables, sauerkraut, and fermented fruits, as well as fermented beverages like kombucha (a fermented beverage usually made from green or black tea). They are also found in sourdough baked goods, and while these bacteria assist in the digestion of sourdough baked goods, they are killed by the heat of the baking process so there are none remaining in the final product. You may still benefit from the easier-to-digest final baked good, however.

You'll also see strains of *Bifidobacteria* listed on an ingredient label as *B. bifidum, B. breve, B. infantis,* and so on. These probiotics tend to have an affinity for the large intestines. There are approximately seven times as many *Bifidobacteria* than *Lactobacilli* present in a healthy adult gut. Newborn babies who have been breastfed tend to have an especially large number of these bacteria in their gastrointestinal tract, which helps them to fight off harmful childhood infections. They are strong immune boosters that tend to be found in yogurt, fermented vegetables, sauerkraut, and kombucha.

You may also see other strains such as *Saccharomyces boulardii* (*S. boulardii*), which is a beneficial type of yeast and, as such, is included among probiotics. They are different from the varieties of yeast that cause yeast infections, so there is no concern about them contributing to a yeast infection if you have one.

REASONS TO BOOST THE GOOD BUGS IN YOUR MICROBIOME

If you haven't been living in a cave or somewhere in the wilderness for the last several years, you've probably noticed that wherever you look on television, online, magazines, and in grocery and health food stores probiotics have popped up in products everywhere. As the exciting research about microbiomes and the importance of maintaining a healthy microbial balance appears, so do probiotic products. So, you may be wondering, what's all the fuss about probiotics? Here are some of the benefits of probiotics as well as reasons for incorporating more of them in your diet and boosting their ability to proliferate in your gut:[6,7]

1. Probiotics help restore microbial balance after it has been disrupted due to antibiotic use or poor food choices.
2. Probiotics create compounds that destroy harmful bacteria.
3. Probiotics strengthen immunity in the gut to bolster the body's own immune response.
4. They decrease inflammation in the gut, which in turn helps to reduce inflammation throughout the body.
5. Probiotics help to program the immune system, yielding more balanced immune responses.
6. They improve the mucosal barrier in the gut and its functioning to prevent harmful infections from entering the body. Some probiotics seem to prevent the ability of harmful bacteria, including *H. pylori,* from adhering to the walls of the GI tract, thereby preventing the ability of the harmful microbes to survive.
7. Probiotics help to regulate genetic expression for health.
8. They create valuable nutrients needed by the body for strong immune health and overall health.

9. They prevent harmful microbes from adhering to various locations in the body, such as in the gut wall.

10. Bacteria in the *Lactobacillus* genus have been found to reinforce the protective functions in the stomach and GI tract by maintaining bacterial balance.

The simple addition of more probiotic-rich food or probiotic supplements can offer a wealth of health advantages.

CAN TAKING PROBIOTICS WITH ANTIBIOTICS HELP?

If you're like most people, you're probably familiar with some of the more immediate side-effects of taking antibiotic drugs, including GI distress, intestinal bacterial overgrowth, and diarrhea.

Antibiotics cause diarrhea and other gastrointestinal issues because they indiscriminately kill harmful and beneficial bacteria alike. Taking probiotic supplements during and after a course of antibiotics can help reduce the damage to the gut microbiome and the GI symptoms, and may prevent opportunistic infections like *C. diff.* that some people experience while taking antibiotics. Diarrhea, one of the common symptoms of antibiotic use, is also one of the main symptoms of *C. diff* infections.

Plentiful amounts of research support the use of probiotics alongside antibiotics. In a Finnish study, researchers found a correlation between a higher dose of probiotics and a lowered incidence and duration of diarrhea experienced by people taking antibiotic drugs. Study participants taking probiotic supplements also had fewer fevers, abdominal pain, and bloating.[8]

In a study published in *JAMA: The Journal of the American Medical Association,* researchers found that a probiotic supplement containing *Lactobacillus, Bifidobacterium, Saccharomyces, Streptococcus, Enterococcus,* or *Bacillus* bacteria was helpful in overcoming antibiotic-related symptoms.[9] A separate Swedish study found that *Lactobacillus plantarum* (*L. plantarum*) was also helpful when taken as a supplement during antibiotic treatment.[10]

Taking probiotics whenever you're following a course of antibiotics isn't just beneficial to reduce the side effects of antibiotics, they can provide additional protection against infectious diseases as well. Because many antibiotics are waning in their effectiveness against harmful microbes, probiotics provide an extra line of defense against harmful infectious diseases. While the use of probiotics as a weapon against infectious disease is fairly novel, a growing body of research shows that probiotics offer antibacterial, antifungal, and antiviral support for your body as well as the well-documented other health benefits to your body.

PROBIOTICS TO THE RESCUE

We already know that our immune system has a wealth of strategies and warriors against infectious disease, but we also know that sometimes our immune system needs a boost. Can you imagine a whole army of bacteria showing up as extra troops in the battle against infectious disease? Increasing amounts of research are showing us that probiotic bacteria (and to a lesser extent, some beneficial yeasts) can not only support your immune system to ensure your health, but can actually wage war against specific harmful invaders too.

Part of their anti-infectious magic lies in the fact that probiotics compete with harmful, disease-causing microbes for space, nutrients, and even the ability to attach to human hosts, according to research.[11] It turns out that probiotics thrive at the expense of harmful microbes, like the viruses behind some of our common illnesses, causing these viruses to die. A reduction in symptoms and illness are the side effects of their battle. You won't find that side effect on the pages-long list of side effects for drugs.[12]

What's more, Iranian researchers discovered that at least one type of probiotic known as *Lactobacillus rhamnosus* (*L. rhamnosus*) enhanced the body's ability to produce the immune cells known as macrophages.[13] As you may recall from our discussion in chapter 1, macrophages are fairly large cells compared to other bodily cells. They engulf harmful microbes and destroy them before they can settle further into the body and cause disease. Boosting production of these immune system cells is a huge benefit in arming your body against infectious diseases.

Even if some bacteria or viruses survive the attack of the macrophages, exciting research published in the journal *Clinical and Experimental Immunology* found that the probiotics *L. plantarum* and *Lactobacillus paracasei* (*L. paracasei*) may also boost the body's production of killer T-cells that act as another line of defense against harmful invaders.[14]

Some of the Probiotic Superstars

There are many different strains of probiotics, but to date, some of the ones that stand out as the superstars that boost the immune system and bolster our defenses against infectious diseases include *Bifidobacterium bifidum* (*B. bifidum*), *Lactobacillus brevis* (*L. brevis*), *Lactobacillus casei* (*L. casei*), *Lactobacillus gasseri* (*L. gasseri*), *L. paracasei*, *L. plantarum*, and *L. rhamnosus*. Of course, there are many other great probiotics and as research continues to pour in about the antibacterial, antifungal, and antiviral strains of specific probiotic strains, many others may be added to the list.

The best way to ensure a strong immune system against a range of microbial threats is to eat a wide variety of fermented foods with live cultures to ensure diverse strains of probiotics in your daily diet. Additionally, supplementing with a broad-spectrum, high quality probiotic supplement from a reputable company may also be helpful. Unfortunately, finding one that fits the bill might take a bit of effort as there are unscrupulous companies producing these types of products, like in any industry.

Of course, you'll want to read the label to ensure that any of the specific strains above that might be beneficial for your particular health needs are found in the product you select. Many broad-spectrum probiotic supplements contain: *Bifidobacterium breve* (*B. breve*), *B. bifidum*, *Bifidobacterium infantis* (*B. infantis*), *Bifidobacterium lactis* (*B. lactis*), *Bifidobacterium longus* (*B. longus*), *Lactobacillus acidophilus* (*L. acidophilus*), *Lactobacillus Bulgaricus* (*L. Bulgaricus*), *L. paracasei*, *L. plantarum*, *L. rhamnosus*, *Propionibacterium freudenreichi* (*P. freudenreichi*), and *Streptococcus thermophilus* (*S. thermophilus*).

It's not necessary for a supplement to contain all of these strains, nor does a product that purports to contain all of these strains ensure that they will be found within the product, in the numbers of cultures claimed, or that they are indeed live. That's why it is also imperative to consider other factors when purchasing probiotic supplements.

What is the reputation of the company manufacturing the probiotic product? Due to the growing popularity of probiotics, many companies are jumping on the bandwagon to profit from the trend. While there is nothing inherently wrong with a start-up company, you'll want to know the company is committed to third-party proof that their product claims are valid. Too many companies are offering the world but may not deliver on the claims.

By the time most probiotic products get to you, they have already gone through the manufacturing, transportation, and distribution processes, and may have even sat on the shelves of grocery stores, health food stores, or pharmacies for some time before you bring the product home for use. It is important to know that probiotics are measured in colony forming units, or CFU, which is the number of live bacteria per milliliter. Product labels typically claim one to fifty billion CFU of specific strains of probiotics. Some companies list the CFU "at the time of manufacture" while others list the number at the end of the shelf life of the product. Since probiotic numbers are constantly in a state of decline, the latter number is more accurate and better reflects the actual number of probiotics you may be getting. Of course, reading the lower number on the label might not sound as impressive, but the number of probiotic cultures "at the time of manufacture" is somewhat misleading to consumers. Most people benefit from at least one billion CFU but some health conditions would benefit from higher doses. There are no hard and fast rules as this is entirely an emerging field of natural medicine. Storage in a refrigerator also helps to prolong their shelf life.

Ideally, choose a product that contains both *Bifidobacterium* and *Lactobacillus* strains because the former are more likely to inoculate the large intestine while the latter are more likely to inoculate the small intestine. You'll get better results by improving the microbial balance in both the large and small intestines.

Check the product expiration date as it may give you an idea as to how long the probiotic supplement has been sitting in a manufacturing facility, distribution warehouse, or retailer's store. If it's close to the expiration date, the product likely has far fewer live bacteria than the number of CFU reported on the label.

If you suffer from a corn, gluten, milk, soy, wheat, or another allergy, be sure to check the label. Many probiotics are manufactured in facilities where other products are packaged so there is the potential for cross-contamination. Many probiotics, especially *Lactobacillus* strains, are derived from dairy sources so you'll especially want to ensure it is a dairy-free product if you have an allergy to dairy products.

There's no product that is better than all the others because there's no one-size-fits-all probiotic supplement. You'll want one that is best suited for your health needs. If the product is intended for a child, you'll want one formulated for a child, or conversely, if the product is intended for a senior, then choose one formulated for seniors. Of course, consider health issues, for which I will share some of the exciting research below to help you select a product that contains the most important, research-supported strains for any health issues you may be dealing with. For example, research has shown that *H. pylori* infections that are often implicated in ulcers tend to respond to *Bifidobacterium* and *Saccharomyces* strains, while vaginal infections seem to respond better to *L. rhamnosus,* according to our current knowledge of probiotics.

Whether you're dealing with cold viruses, cold sores (caused by the herpes virus), or a more serious bacterial, fungal, or viral infection, fermented foods and probiotics are demonstrating their impressive capacity in a growing body of research.

A study published in the *British Journal of Nutrition* found that consumption of probiotic-containing yogurt reduced the frequency with which elderly people suffered from respiratory infections and cut the duration of the infections by one and a half days compared to the placebo group.[15] The yogurt used in the study contained *Lactobacillus casei* probiotics.

In a study published in the *European Journal of Nutrition* found that *L. plantarum* and *L. paracasei* reduced the risk of catching the common cold, reduced severity of cold symptoms, and shortened its duration by approximately two and a half days. Considering that the prevention of the common cold has eluded drug companies, this is a noteworthy accomplishment.[16]

Research in the *Journal of Applied Microbiology* also found that probiotics helped to prevent and speed the healing of ear and respiratory infections.[17]

Probiotics are demonstrating their antiviral potential in other conditions as well, including in the prevention and treatment of the herpes simplex virus that is linked to cold sores. Italian researchers found that the probiotic *Lactobacillus brevis* demonstrated antiviral activity against the herpes simplex virus by preventing its ability to multiply.[18] The probiotic *L. plantarum* also demonstrated antiviral activity against the herpes simplex virus.[19]

The future of medicine likely includes the increasing use of a wide variety of probiotics, even within the therapeutic strategy for treating many serious illnesses, like genital herpes or HIV. In a preliminary animal study, scientists found that the probiotics *L. plantarum* and *S. thermophilus* inhibited the viruses linked to influenza, genital herpes, and HIV by preventing them from reproducing.[20] Since viruses rely on reproduction to survive, these probiotics may hold promise for the prevention and early treatment of viral conditions.

Probiotics are demonstrating promise against fungal infections, namely *C. albicans,* as well. While *Candida* is often called a yeast infection, it is a fungal infection that can attack the GI tract, mucous membranes of the mouth, or vagina. In a small study published in the journal *Mycopathologia,* researchers found that yogurt consumption reduced *Candida* infections in women.[21]

Almost every day new studies showcase the exciting findings of scientists around the world who are finding that probiotics are demonstrating antibacterial, antiviral, and antifungal effects against a wide range of conditions. And, the list of conditions in which probiotics may be helpful as a direct method of treatment continues to grow.

PROBIOTICS REGULATE SOMETIMES DEADLY IMMUNE OVERACTIVITY

Infections like bacterial and viral illnesses often hijack the body's powerful immune response, make our immune system work overtime, and cause inflammatory damage to healthy cells and tissues. Known as a "cytokine storm," this infection-induced immune system response is often behind severe symptoms and an increased risk of death.

Exciting new research in the field of probiotics is showing these beneficial microbes offer yet another benefit for our health as it seems they may help to regulate these cytokine storms while also reducing damaging inflammation to healthy bodily tissues. A study published in the *Journal of the American College of Nutrition* found that supplementation with the two probiotic strains the researchers tested— *L. gasseri* and *B. bifidum* both resulted in reduced cytokine activity and inflammation.[22]

Ways to Support Your Microbiome

The first step in restoring a healthy gut microbiome is to eliminate or reduce the factors that destroy beneficial microbes, while boosting the foods and lifestyle practices that support a healthy microbiome. Some of these things include:

- Stop using toxic antibacterial soaps, cleaning products, and hand sanitizers—of course, there are healthier options than those that contain toxic triclosan or other harmful chemicals.
- Use antibiotics only when prescribed for bacterial infections, not colds and flu that are caused by viruses.
- Use antibiotics as described for the full course of treatment. If your doctor prescribed antibiotics for one week, use them for the full week. (And, please do not flush antibiotics into the water supply where they can disrupt delicate ecosystems.)
- Switch to natural personal care products since they are less likely to damage the microbiome on our skin.
- Switch to natural cleaning products devoid of toxic fragrances or harsh solvents.
- Switch to organic foods wherever possible. While many people believe "certified organic" is the way to go, I believe costly government-run certification programs are actually harmful to many small-scale farmers and prefer to recommend produce that is grown from trustworthy local farmers in your area.
- Increase your intake of prebiotic-rich foods.
- Increase your intake of fermented foods like sauerkraut, kimchi, yogurt, and fermented pickles.
- Reduce the sugar intake in your diet in favor of fruit, since the fiber and sugar in fruit act as prebiotics (food for probiotics) and therefore help increase quantities of probiotics.
- Avoid eating excessive amounts of fatty and processed meats as they can quickly throw off the microbial balance in favor of inflammatory types.

- Incorporate wild foods into your diet. Wild foods tend to be nutrient-dense and many contain prebiotics, and some even contain beneficial microbes. Of course, choose only wild foods that you are completely confident you have correctly identified.
- Drink sufficient water since it helps to ensure healthy bowel movements that also transport harmful microbes out of the body once they have been killed by beneficial varieties.

RAMPING UP YOUR BENEFICIAL MICROBES

Most people grab yogurt when they want to give their probiotics a boost. While yogurt may be a good way to boost two or three strains of beneficial bacteria, it's not necessarily the only, or even the best way.

There are many other foods that contain a greater diversity of probiotics in higher numbers than yogurt. Some of these foods include: naturally-fermented vegetables like pickles, kimchi (a spicy Korean condiment), and sauerkraut; kombucha (naturally fermented tea); miso (fermented soy, chickpea, or rice that is often used in soups); and kefir (pronounced ke-FEER), which is a cultured milk or juice product similar to yogurt, but typically thinner.

There are many other fermented foods and it is worth experimenting to find the ones you like best as well as to eat a diverse range of them to ensure probiotic diversity as well.

While some people include sourdough breads among probiotic-rich foods, any beneficial bacteria are killed during the baking process. That doesn't mean that artisanal sourdough bread isn't superior to commercially leavened bread, it simply is not a source of probiotics. It is still more digestible than other types of breads and worth consuming.

Of course, if you enjoy yogurt, it's worth including in your diet. There are also many plant-based types of yogurts, many of which contain live cultures. Some plant-based yogurts include almond, cashew, coconut, and soy.

Regardless of which type of fermented foods you select, make sure they contain "live cultures;" this is usually documented on the label. Alternatively, the label may say "unpasteurized" or "naturally fermented," all of which are signs that the product you selected is likely to contain probiotics. Of course, exposure to heat or other factors can reduce their numbers, so live cultures are not guaranteed. To learn more about fermented foods or how to make them, check out my book *The Cultured Cook.*

Supplementation with either probiotic powder, which can be added to juice or water, or probiotic capsules can also be a great way to boost the probiotics in your diet and body.

There's another little-known way to boost probiotics in your body: eat foods that act as food for probiotics.

Eating more probiotic-rich food and popping supplements aren't the only ways to increase the populations of beneficial microbes in your intestines. One of the best ways to do so is to add more foods to your diet that beneficial microbes thrive on, which are sometimes referred to as prebiotics or prebiotic foods. Most plant-based foods act as prebiotics, but fruits are particularly good. Doing so helps to increase their numbers, which in turn, offers peripheral benefits to your health and immunity.

While probiotics are largely used as a broad-scale health-booster and, to date, the medical profession has largely ignored the ever-growing amount of research to support the use of specific probiotics to target infectious disease conditions, I believe we are on the cusp of discovering this little-known way to prevent or treat infectious diseases, including ones that are escaping our so-called best medicines, antibiotics. As antibiotics are winding down their role in the treatment of infectious disease, probiotics are rising to the occasion to potentially become among the new best practices for the treatment of bacterial, fungal, and viral diseases. Learn more in my book *Super-Powered Immunity Starts in the Gut.*

5
Mushrooms

Experience the Magic of Fungi for
Super-Powered Immunity

When it comes to building super-powered immunity and fighting infectious microbes, mushrooms really can impart their magic. No, I'm not referring to magic mushrooms with their hallucinogenic properties, some of the best immune-builders are readily available mushrooms. The real magical power of mushrooms like reishi, chaga, lion's mane, turkey tail, and shiitake lay in their ability to supercharge your immune system. Much maligned and often shunned simply for looking weird and growing in unusual places, edible mushrooms are potent medicines and delicious additions to a healthy diet that can supercharge your immune system.

Mushrooms have been used as medicine for thousands of years, particularly among Chinese, Egyptian, Greek, Mexican, and Roman cultures.[1] In 1991, the medical journal the *Lancet* reported a discovery of a well-preserved man's body that was termed the "Ice Man" since his body had been found frozen in ice. Determined to be 5,300 years old, the man's effects were preserved alongside his body and found to include a birch fungus believed to have been his medicine to treat intestinal parasites.[2]

There are an estimated fourteen to twenty-two thousand species of mushrooms worldwide, of which many are edible and medicinal, offering beneficial nutrients or therapeutic compounds.[3] Of course, not all mushrooms are edible and some are poisonous, so if you're foraging for mushrooms to boost your immune system, you'll want to work with a knowledgeable and experienced guide.

A growing body of medical and clinical research continues to reveal the immune-boosting power of mushrooms like reishi, chaga, lion's mane, turkey tail, and shiitake. In this chapter, you'll also learn how to get more of these immune-boosting superstars into your diet and how to choose the best mushrooms for your specific needs.

In this chapter, you'll discover:

- The mushroom that has the widest antiviral activity;
- The mushroom that contains four hundred therapeutic compounds that can be used to help build super-powered immunity;
- The mushroom that increases killer cells in the body while also regulating the immune system;
- The mushroom that has demonstrated antiviral activity against the viruses that cause hepatitis B and HIV;
- The mushroom that research shows has antibacterial activity against *E. coli,* a bacterium that causes food-poisoning; and
- The mushrooms that have demonstrated effectiveness against yeast infections.

Chaga
(*Inonotus obliquus*)

The Finnish name of this mushroom, cancer polypore, provides some insight into the application for which this mushroom is primarily known—cancer.[4] Chaga mushrooms are also sometimes called chaga conk or birch mushrooms because the black fungus grows on birch trees, although they occasionally also grow on alder trees. Weighing up to approximately four and a half pounds (two kilograms), they can also grow to over two yards (two meters) in size.

While chaga contains more than two hundred constituents, including many medicinal ones, several compounds in particular, including polyphenols, betulin, and betulinic acid, have been shown to offer potent therapeutic benefits.[5] Polyphenols are powerful antioxidants that destroy harmful free radicals. In one study, researchers found that chaga reduced the oxidative stress in immune cells known as lymphocytes.[6] Other research found that chaga also inhibits genetic damage in these immune cells.[7]

Cordyceps
(Ophiocordyceps sinensis
syn. Clonorchis sinensis)

Not technically considered a mushroom, cordyceps is often grouped with mushrooms for ease of sharing information, so I have included it here. It is a type of fungus that grows in high altitudes in the Tibetan Plateau and neighboring regions, including China, Nepal, Tibet, and India. Also known as Chinese caterpillar mushroom, or winter worm, it is also found in other areas outside of China. Cordyceps contains active therapeutic compounds known as polysaccharides, cordycepin, and cordycepic acid.

Research found that eight weeks of supplementation with an extract of cordyceps increased natural killer cell activity, thereby boosting immune response while also regulating the immune system.[8] Other studies found that cordyceps increased immunocyte activity and immunoglobulin production.[9]

Lion's Mane
(Hericium erinaceus)

The mushroom known as lion's mane, after its white, fur-like appearance, is demonstrating significant immune system benefits. A growing body of research shows that consumption of lion's mane can improve gut health,[10] which as you know is a foundation for healthy immunity.

Maitake
(*Grifola frondose*)

Both a culinary and medicinal mushroom, maitake has been found to contain a compound known as proteoglucan, which is associated with its immune-stimulating effects.[11]

In both laboratory and animal studies, research shows that polysaccharides found in maitake mushrooms have demonstrated antiviral activity against both hepatitis B viruses and HIV.[12]

Oyster
(*Pleurotus ostreatus* and *Pleurotus florida*)

There are several species of oyster mushrooms, which are primarily known for their culinary uses, but research shows that these delicious mushrooms may also improve immune health. Readily available in grocery stores and at farmer's markets, oyster mushrooms contain many nutrients and therapeutic compounds, including protein, vitamin C, iron, potassium, copper, and zinc, all of which are important for strong immunity, particularly the vitamin C and zinc.[13]

Most known for their ability to reduce cholesterol levels similarly to statin drugs as well as for their anticancer and antitumor ability, oyster mushrooms also demonstrate antimicrobial properties. They showed antibiotic activity against the bacteria *Micrococcus luteus, S. aureus,* and *Bacillus mycoides.* The mushrooms also demonstrate activity against the aggressive mold known as *Aspergillis niger,* which can cause aspergillosis lung disease, particularly in those with weak immune systems. Oyster mushrooms inhibit hepatitis C virus and may be beneficial against HIV as well.[14]

Reishi
(*Ganoderma lucidum*)

Reishi, or *ling zhi,* which means "spirit plant" or "tree of life mushroom" in Chinese, has rightfully gained popularity for its many healing properties, including boosting the immune system, relaxing muscles and the nervous system, protecting the respiratory tract, and much more.[15]

Reishi's immune-supporting properties alone make it an excellent mushroom to incorporate into your diet or supplement regime on a regular basis. Animal research shows that reishi enhanced immune cells like interleukin-1 and white blood cells created in the bone marrow. It also demonstrates broad antibacterial and antiviral properties largely due to its ability to activate the immune system. Tea made from reishi showed activity against *Bacillus, Micrococcus, Streptococcus,* and *Staphylococcus* bacteria. Reishi has even demonstrated anti-HIV activity both in laboratory and human studies.[16]

Shiitake
(*Lentinula edodes*)

Commonly found in Japanese cuisine, shiitake is a unique mushroom with a magical effect on the immune system. According to research published in the *Journal of the American College of Nutrition,* those who regularly ate shiitake mushrooms were rewarded with improved immunity—better immune cell activation and higher levels of an immune system warrior known as immunoglobulin A (also referred to as IgA). The study authors also concluded that changes observed in other immunity markers suggested a possible reduction in inflammation linked to the consumption of the mushrooms.[17]

Shiitake mushrooms are native to eastern Asia but they are one of the most readily available mushrooms due to their increasing popularity. They are frequently found in the produce section of many grocery stores. Their rich, smoky flavor complements many types of cuisine, as well as meat, poultry, or vegetarian dishes alike.

Turkey Tail
(*Trametes versicolor,*
Coriolus versicolor, and *Polyporous versicolor*)

Fan-shaped, with curved stripes, this mushroom resembles a turkey tail, which has led to its name. Turkey tail mushroom is considered by experts as one of the most important medicinal mushrooms in the world, in part due to its anticancer and antitumor properties that are supported with research.

A water-soluble protein found in turkey tail, known as polysaccharide krestin (PSK) boosts interferon production. It also has antiviral properties and has even been found to inhibit HIV. Polysaccharide peptide (PSP), another compound found in turkey tail, has immune-stimulating properties and prevents immune system decline.[18]

Tea made with turkey tail mushroom demonstrates antibacterial activity against *S. aureus, P. aeruginosa, E. coli, K. pneumoniae, Staphylococcus albus, Streptococcus salivarius,* and *Salmonella paratyphi.* Turkey tail tea is also helpful against *Vibrio cholerae* and *Shigella paradysenteria,* more likely to be encountered in developing countries.[19]

If that isn't enough reason to love turkey tail, a year-long study of turkey tail's impact on HPV found that it resulted in a 72 percent decrease in cervical dysplasia lesions linked to the virus.[20] Other research showed that turkey tail is also active against malaria. Additionally, the mushroom shows antifungal and antiparasitic activity.[21]

HEALING WITH MUSHROOMS

Mushrooms are delicious and versatile. They can easily take the place of meat in any meal (think portobello instead of steak) and are excellent additions to soups, stews, and curries. They also lend a rich flavor to gravies and support a vegan or vegetarian lifestyle.

A wide variety of edible mushrooms can be found in grocery stores, health food stores, and many farmers' markets. Purchasing from these retailers takes the risk out of eating mushrooms because they have been harvested by knowledgeable "shroomers" who understand the difference between edible and inedible, or poisonous, varieties. It also gives you an opportunity to try health-enhancing mushrooms that may not be indigenous to where you live.

Some of these mushrooms are available as powders that you can add to water to make a tea, soup, stew, or other dishes. I recommend adding it after you finish cooking to ensure the full nutritional and medicinal value of the mushrooms.

Additionally, many of these mushrooms are available as alcohol-based extracts in which the medicinal properties of the mushrooms are extracted and made bioavailable. Follow package instructions for the product you select. Of course, avoid alcohol preparations if you are an alcoholic, are pregnant or nursing, or have liver disease, or with children. Consult the product package for other potential contraindications.

While wildcrafting (wandering the woods and harvesting mushrooms straight from Mother Nature) is enjoyable and fulfilling, it is best left to mushroom experts who can identify species accurately and who will practice sustainable harvesting methods that won't damage the long-term viability of the mushroom ecosystem.

If you decide you want to wildcraft mushrooms, enroll yourself in a credible, hands-on workshop with an experienced mycologist that brings you into direct contact with the mushroom varieties in your area. Relying on an illustrated book is not enough to fully understand the complex and strangely beautiful world of these fantastic fungi; however, it is a great way to learn more about these powerful and magical forest dwellers.

I recommend *The Fungal Pharmacy: The Complete Guide to Medicinal Mushrooms & Lichens of North America* by registered herbalist Robert Rogers (American Herbalists Guild). I cannot speak highly enough of this brilliant masterpiece, which has become the bible of medicinal mushrooms among shroomers and natural medicine practitioners alike.

Mushrooms for Common Microbial Conditions[22]

While there are many mushrooms that boost immunity and have specific antibacterial, antifungal, and antiviral effects, the following information contains some of the most readily available mushrooms that also demonstrated their effectiveness in studies against certain microbes. There are many other mushrooms that have demonstrated activity against these bacteria, fungi, and viruses; however, this table includes only those mushrooms discussed in this chapter, which I've selected for their readily available nature.

Additionally, many other mushrooms have demonstrated their ability to inhibit many other microbes, but they are beyond the scope of this chapter. For much more detailed research-supported information about which mushrooms are best for specific microbes, consult *The Fungal Pharmacy,* which includes a five-page chart of research-supported mushrooms and their effectiveness against many other infectious microbes, as well as detailed information on some lesser-known mushrooms and their uses for these conditions.

Bacteria

Bacillus species: This group includes many different species of gram-positive, rod-shaped bacteria that are involved in food poisoning, wound infections, or blood infections (sepsis), among other health conditions, depending on the species involved.[23] Two of the mushrooms that have demonstrated activity against *Bacillus* include lion's mane and oyster.

Escherichia coli: More commonly known as *E. coli,* this group of bacteria are normally harmless and live in the intestines of humans and animals, but certain strains found in contaminated water or food can cause food poisoning and severe kidney disease.[24] Oyster mushrooms have demonstrated activity against *E. coli* bacteria.

Mycobacterium tuberculosis: The bacteria behind one of the oldest human afflictions, tuberculosis, *M. tuberculosis,* still impact millions of people on the planet every year.[25] Maitake mushrooms have demonstrated activity against these bacteria.

Pseudomonas species: A group of bacteria that live in soil and water, *Pseudomonas* infections can affect different parts of the body. The most common type, *P. aeruginosa,* primarily inhabit pools, hot tubs, and contact lenses, and are therefore often behind infections acquired from these sources.[26] Oyster mushrooms have demonstrated activity against these bacteria.

Fungi

Aspergillus: A common mold found in hay, compost, soil, and basements, these microorganisms have may different species that can impact human health, causing sinus or respiratory infections, among other issues.[27] Lion's mane, maitake, and oyster mushrooms have all demonstrated antifungal activity against *Aspergillus.*

Candida albicans: While *C. albicans* are readily found in the human microbiome, it is the most common fungal species that can cause illness by infecting any or all of the gut, mouth, or vaginal areas.[28] Lion's mane and maitake mushrooms have demonstrated activity against *Candida* microorganisms.

Viruses

HIV: HIV is the sexually-transmitted, potentially life-threatening disease that causes acquired immunodeficiency disease (AIDS).[29] Both maitake and oyster mushrooms have demonstrated activity against HIV.

6

Habits That Hurt, Habits That Help

The things we do on a daily basis either contribute to a strong immune system or they thwart our body's best ability to keep us healthy. We can use all the natural or synthetic medicines that are best suited for fighting illness but it's important to address other issues that may be interfering with keeping our body strong and healthy.

It probably doesn't need to be stated that stress is one of the worst things that deplete the immune system as most people have seen the damaging effects of stress firsthand. Perhaps you've gotten a cold when you were under a lot of stress? Or perhaps you experienced a setback with another health problem when unexpected stress came along? Regardless, it's important to understand the impact of stress and, more importantly, how to reduce the effects of stress to keep your immune system strong and healthy.

STRESS MANAGEMENT

We tend to think of stress as the enemy, but some stress is actually ben-eficial when it comes to the health of our immune system. According to research published in the journal *Immunologic Research,* short-term stress lasting for only minutes or hours actually improves wound healing, as well as the body's ability to fight infections and tumors. However, excessive amounts or long-term stress can have destructive consequences by suppressing the immune response and worsening immune system diseases.[1]

Research published in *Current Opinions in Psychology* indicates that psychological stress can impair the immune system and its ability to function properly, having different effects depending on whether the stress is acute (short-lived) or chronic (long-term). The journal authors explain the impact of stress on the immune system:

> During acute stress lasting a matter of minutes, certain kinds of cells are mobilized into the bloodstream, potentially preparing the body for injury or infection during "fight or flight." Acute stress also increases blood levels of pro-inflammatory cytokines. Chronic stress lasting from days to years, like acute stress, is associated with higher levels of pro-inflammatory cytokines, but with potentially different health consequences. Inflammation is a necessary short-term response for eliminating pathogens and initiating healing, but chronic, systemic inflammation represents dysregulation of the immune system and increases risk for chronic diseases, including atherosclerosis and frailty. Another consequence of chronic stress is activation of latent viruses. Latent virus activation can reflect the loss of immunological control over the virus, and frequent activation can cause wear-and-tear on the immune system.[2,3]

While stress may sometimes feel overwhelming and impossible to avoid, there are typically many options to reduce stress load or to alleviate the pressure buildup of excessive stress, thereby reducing any possible damage to the immune system.

Body Aches from a Virus?
What to Do for Relief

So, you've caught a flu bug or other virus? Body aches may feel awful but they are a sign that your immune system has actively engaged the virus, battling to overcome it. That doesn't mean you need to suffer unnecessarily though.

Adding a half cup of Epsom salts to your bath water not only relaxes your aching muscles, reducing any discomfort you may be feeling, it also helps to ensure a relaxing and restorative night's sleep, which is critical to maintaining a healthy immune system. And, as you learned in chapter 2, magnesium is needed to ensure that the super-immunity vitamin, Vitamin D, is absorbed. Magnesium is Nature's relaxant, meaning it can help alleviate the stress and muscle tightness that also comes along with being sick.

Add five to eight drops each of eucalyptus and lavender essential oils to your magnesium-infused bath water to further boost its pain-alleviating and healing benefits. The eucalyptus will open your sinuses to alleviate sinus pressure and pain, as well as reduce the discomfort of bodily aches, while the lavender relaxes and soothes your achy muscles and prepares you for a restful night's sleep.

Strategies That Work

There are many ways to cope with stress and strengthen your body's immune system. It probably won't come as a surprise to you that the same things that alleviate stress also help to keep the immune system strong. So, to avoid duplication, I've compiled many of the best habits to adopt for both purposes and for the end goal of alleviating the damaging effects of stress while also strengthening your immune system against infectious diseases.

Don't Skip Meals

Low blood sugar is a serious stress to the body that results in a cascade of stress hormones. While an occasional boost of these hormones might be fine, over time this chronic stressor can actually result in massive swings in blood sugar levels that can deplete the body and contribute to chronic health issues. Remember: your body is fueled by the slow and steady release of natural sugars from having broken down food into its primary components, one of which is sugar. As a result, it is important to eat every few hours to ensure your body has enough energy to effectively perform its many functions, and to avoid fluctuations in stress hormones that cause energy depletion and mood swings and challenge our ability to cope with stress. Don't be tempted to eat something sugary to raise your blood sugar levels. It quickly results in plummeting blood sugar levels that further stress the body and may deplete the immune system.

Eat a High Fiber Diet

You may be wondering how fiber can help alleviate stress. In addition to eating every few hours to ensure that your body has an adequate supply of energy, eating a diet that is high in fiber can also ensure that blood sugar is released slowly and is sustained over hours.

To help you get started boosting your fiber intake, enjoy a bowl of high-fiber oatmeal for breakfast, sprinkle flax or hempseeds on your cereal, add a can of beans to your next soup or stew, add chickpeas to your next rice bowl or atop a salad, and thicken your next smoothie with a tablespoon of chia seeds (drink it up quickly or it will turn to pudding).

Say No to People Who Steal Your Energy

We all have people in our lives who sap our energy. While it may not be possible to eliminate all of these energy thieves, it can be surprising how easy it is to simply take some time out from them or to set stricter boundaries about how your time is spent.

Make a list of the people in your life who sap your strength and create stress in your life. Take an honest assessment of which relationships may be one-sided or who you could see less frequently. Life is short. Surround yourself with people who bring out the best possible you, not stress you out constantly. Of course, everyone is negative or causes stress to others sometimes, it's just all about finding a compassionate balance you can live with.

Take a Vitamin B-Complex and Vitamin C Supplement

These nutrients are depleted during times of high stress, which, of course, also includes fighting infection. Additionally, they are not stored in the body so it is imperative to obtain adequate amounts from food and supplements every day to ensure your brain has sufficient energy to function properly.

Without adequate B-complex vitamins we become susceptible to stress, depression, and irritability. Our bodies deplete high amounts of vitamin C when we're stressed, yet this essential nutrient is needed to fight free radicals that could otherwise damage the brain. B vitamins are largely found in brown rice, root vegetables, citrus fruit, strawberries, cantaloupe, kale, and green vegetables. Supplement with a 50 to 100 milligram B-complex supplement on a daily basis (some of these vitamins are measured in mcg, so 50 to 100 micrograms in these cases).

Vitamin C is found in oranges, lemons, grapefruit, limes, pomegranates, strawberries, black currants, spinach, beet greens, tomatoes, sprouts, and red peppers. Most nutrition experts recommend a 500 milligram ascorbic acid or calcium ascorbate (both of which are natural forms of vitamin C) supplement as a daily minimum.

Meditate or Breathe Deeply

Research in the medical journal *Psychiatry Research* shows that meditation affects the flow of blood to the brain and alters brain activity. Using MRI technology, researchers conducted brain scans before starting, during, and after meditation stopped. They found that four regions of the brain were affected during meditation and that meditation improved blood flow to the brain. Some of the brain changes continued even after meditation stopped.[4]

Just Say No

You may not have to do every task on your to-do list, handle everyone's chores or needs, respond to every message, or accept every social invitation. Obviously, you can't say no to your most pressing tasks, but you can itemize them and prioritize those that must be done, those that might need to be done, and those that are not necessities.

Remove tasks from your list that you really don't need to do. Whether it's your in-laws' request for you to cook dinner or a social visit that feels more obligatory than enjoyable, you can simply say no. You deserve peaceful, quality time devoted to reducing stress.

Ask for Help

Don't try to do everything yourself. Ask your partner, kids, friends, or family to help, or if your financial situation permits, hire someone to help with cleaning, odd jobs, or other items in your home or work that would make life less stressful for you.

Reduce Your Sugar Intake

I know it can be difficult to resist all the sweets during times of stress, but stress-eating may actually be contributing to feeling more stress if you're choosing sweets. Sweets not only impair immune function for hours at a time, making you more vulnerable to colds, flu, or other infectious conditions, they also deplete your reserves for dealing with stress.

And, don't forget that alcohol has a similar effect as white sugar, so it is best to reduce intake to optimize your immune function. In place of sugary snacks, choose high-fiber options like those mentioned above, or high-protein nuts or sunflower or pumpkin seeds, and you'll experience fewer cravings or hunger, making it easier to enjoy a cookie or two but not gorge on the whole stack.

Exercise Your Way to Super-Powered Immunity

We all know exercise is good for us. It's important to get our heart pumping to push blood through our blood vessels and to bring oxygen into the bloodstream. But, it's also important to reduce stress and to keep the immune system functioning optimally. And, cardiovascular activity helps to transport oxygen through your bloodstream.

Research published in the *International Journal of Environmental Research and Public Health* has shown that oxygen, when used therapeutically, has antiviral effects.[5] But, you don't have to go for expensive oxygen therapies to start benefiting from increasing oxygen levels in your body. You can start by getting some cardiovascular activity on a regular basis.

Sleep Your Way to Better Immunity

Research shows that sleep plays a critical role in our overall health, and in influencing our risk of infectious disease. In a study published in the medical journal *Annual Review of Psychology,* researchers found that sleep disturbances, restriction, or insomnia affected both innate and adaptive immunity, which we discussed in chapter 1.

Insufficient sleep also impacts antiviral immune responses and the risk of infectious disease. It can also increase inflammation in the body, which, as you learned earlier, can play a serious role in the outcome of an infectious disease.[6]

Sleep expert and author of *The Promise of Sleep,* William C. Dement, M.D., Ph.D., found in his research that people need at least seven to eight hours of sleep per night on an ongoing basis. He also determined that our bodies keep track of a sleep debt. If we don't get sufficient sleep on a regular basis, it is comparable to making ongoing withdrawals from a sleep account. As with bank accounts, if we always withdraw but never make deposits, we soon run out of money for the things we want or need. In the same way, when it comes to our sleep, we need to make up the lost hours soon afterward or our sleep account continues to go further and further into debt.

But, knowing that insufficient sleep, disturbed sleep, or ongoing difficulty sleeping takes a toll on your immune system doesn't help you if you're struggling with your sleep. Here are some strategies to help you improve the quality and quantity of your sleep. They work best when used on a regular basis over time, so even if you don't get immediate results, I encourage you to stick with them.

- Avoid eating at least three hours before bed as indigestion, bloating, or heartburn can interfere with your ability to fall asleep. Definitely skip the caffeine in the evening or any time after 3:00 in the afternoon if you have difficulty sleeping.
- Get into a regular evening relaxation ritual: dim the lights, stop working, take a bath, or do something relaxing before bedtime.
- Unplug electronic devices or any blue-light emitting appliances like televisions, smartphones, computers, and so on, since the blue light can interfere with sleep cycles. If you need a night light, choose a red bulb since red light doesn't seem to interfere with the body's ability to fall into a deep state of sleep.
- Stop working at least a few hours before bed. Avoid other mentally stimulating activities too close to bedtime.
- Go to sleep at the same time each night. Your body will start to adjust to these patterns, helping you to feel sleepy when your bedtime approaches.
- Alan Hirsch, M.D., an essential oil researcher and author, found that smelling pure lavender calmed the entire nervous system in only a minute, helping people to feel more relaxed and sleepier. Sniff some lavender essential oil or flowers or spray lavender water on your pillowcase (water only since the oil may stain). Be sure to choose organic lavender oil, specifically from *Lavandula angustifolia,* not essential oils of other lavender species that tend to be less

effective, and definitely avoid fragrance oil, since it has no health benefits at all and may contain toxic substances that are detrimental to your health.

Wash Your Hands the Right Way

Most people are well aware that handwashing is one of the best ways to prevent the contraction of viral illnesses like colds, flu, and others. But, using soaps or sanitizers that contain harmful toxic ingredients that can absorb into your bloodstream directly through your skin isn't helpful for your immune system health and will likely deplete the beneficial microbes on the surface of your skin as well.

You're far better off to use a natural soap devoid of toxic chemical ingredients and spend several more seconds washing your hands. As an important bonus, you'll be less likely to contribute to drug resistance and suberbugs that our population will need to contend with for years. That's because many harsh soaps and sanitizers often contain harmful ingredients, like triclosan and others, that are driving microbes to evolve to overcome these chemicals.

It is not necessary to incorporate every strategy mentioned above to reap immune-boosting benefits. Incorporating these strategies into your life isn't meant to be stressful or create tension, but to reduce the immune-damaging effects of stress. In the same way, it is not necessary to eat every immune-supporting food or take every herbal or other remedy outlined earlier, but to gently support your body's ability to ward off harmful infections.

Your body knows it is an incredible creation that has the ability to fight infection and heal itself. It can simply perform its multitude of impressive immune-supporting tasks even more effectively when you reduce the stress in your life as much as possible (remembering some stress is actually beneficial) and give your body additional tools in the form of foods and natural medicines to support your health. And, if you need a reminder as to which remedies to select, be sure to refer back to the section "How to Choose Your Natural Medicines" on page 26.

Your body is far more powerful than you might believe, and it works every second of every day in a diligent effort to fight illness and keep you healthy. Adding some key remedies and strategies will help support it and will be worth the minimal effort.

Notes

CHAPTER 1. UNCOVER YOUR POWERFUL IMMUNE RESPONSE

1. "A Brief Overview of the Immune System," Revere Health website, accessed October 1, 2021.
2. "The Immune System: What Is the Immune System?" Johns Hopkins Medicine website, accessed October 8, 2021.
3. "Common Cold in Children," Stanford Children's Health website, accessed January 27, 2022.
4. "How Does the Immune System Work?" Institute for Quality and Efficiency in Health Care website, accessed November 3, 2021.
5. "How Does the Immune System Work?" Institute for Quality and Efficiency in Health Care website, accessed November 3, 2021.
6. "How Does the Immune System Work?" Institute for Quality and Efficiency in Health Care website, accessed November 3, 2021.
7. Pritish K. Tosh, "What Are Superbugs and How Can I Protect Myself from Infection?" Mayo Clinic website, accessed November 4, 2021.
8. "Biography of Louis Pasteur, French Biologist and Chemist," ThoughtCo. website.
9. "Typhoid Fever and Paratyphoid Fever," Centers for Disease Control and Prevention website, accessed October 7, 2022.
10. "History: Alexander Fleming (1881–1955)," BBC website.
11. "Robert Koch," Wikipedia.
12. Aoife Howard et al., *"Acinetobacter baumannii," Virulence* 3, no. 3 (May 1, 2012): 243–50.

13. Valentina Virginia Ebani et al., "Antimicrobial Activity of Five Essential Oils Against Bacteria and Fungi Responsible for Urinary Tract Infections," *Molecules* 23, no. 7 (July 9, 2018): 1668.

14. N. Rastogi et al., "The Mycobacteria: An Introduction to Nomenclature and Pathogenesis," *Revue Scientifique et Technique* 20, no. 1 (April 2001): 21–54.

15. "Pseudomonas aeruginosa," Science Direct website, accessed February 8, 2022.

16. Tracey A. Taylor and Chandrashekhar G. Unakal, "Staphylococcus Aureus," National Institute of Health's National Library of Medicine website, accessed February 8, 2022.

17. Chris Wodskou, "Bacteria Getting Upper Hand in Antibiotics Arms Race," CBC News website, March 1, 2014.

18. Stephen Harrod Buhner, *Herbal Antibiotics: Natural Alternatives for Treating Drug-Resistant Bacteria* (North Adams, Mass.: Storey Publishing, 2012), 26.

19. Brandon Keim, "Antibiotics Breed Superbugs Faster Than Expected," Wired website, February 11, 2010.

20. "Patients: Information about CRE," Centers for Disease Control website, accessed November 4, 2021.

21. Buhner, *Herbal Antibiotics,* 18.

22. Buhner, *Herbal Antibiotics,* 19.

23. Charles Patrick David, "Medical Definition of RNA Virus," MedicineNet website, accessed December 13, 2021.

24. "Cytomegalovirus (CMV)," WebMD, accessed December 13, 2021.

CHAPTER 2. FOODS AND NUTRIENTS

1. "Vitamins and Minerals," The Nutrition Source, Harvard T.H. Chan School of Public Health website, accessed December 8, 2021.

2. Maria A. Neag et al., "Berberine: Botanical Occurrence, Traditional Uses, Extraction Methods, and Relevance in Cardiovascular, Metabolic, Hepatic, and Renal Disorders," *Frontiers in Pharmacology* 9 (2018): 557.

3. Xizhan Xu et al., "Antidiabetic Effects of Gegen Qinlian Decoction Via the Gut Microbiota Are Attributable to Its Key Ingredient Berberine," *Genomics, Proteomics, and Bioinformatics* 18, no. 6 (December 2020): 721–36.

4. Danyang Song et al., "Biological Properties and Clinical Applications of

Berberine," *Frontiers of Medicine* 14, no. 5 (October 2020): 564–82.

5. Faisal Jamshaid et al., "New Development of Novel Berberine Derivatives Against Bacteria," *Mini Reviews in Medicinal Chemistry* 20, no. 8 (2020): 716–24.

6. Yufei Xie et al., "In Vitro Antifungal Effects of Berberine Against *Candida* spp. in Planktonic and Biofilm Conditions," *Drug Design, Development and Therapy* 14 (January 9, 2020): 87–101.

7. Alicja Warowicka et al., "Antiviral Activity of Berberine," *Archives of Virology* 165, no. 9 (September 2020): 1935–45.

8. Soheil Zorofchian Moghadamtousi et al., "A Review of Antibacterial, Antiviral, and Antifungal Activity of Curcumin," *BioMed Research International* (2014).

9. Moghadamtousi et al., "A Review of Antibacterial, Antiviral, and Antifungal Activity of Curcumin."

10. Su Hyun Mun et al., "Synergistic Antibacterial Effect of Curcumin Against Methicillin-Resistant *Staphylococcus aureus*," *Phytomedicine* 20, no. 8–9 (June 15, 2013): 714–18.

11. Moghadamtousi et al., "A Review of Antibacterial, Antiviral, and Antifungal Activity of Curcumin."

12. Moghadamtousi et al., "A Review of Antibacterial, Antiviral, and Antifungal Activity of Curcumin."

13. Moghadamtousi et al., "A Review of Antibacterial, Antiviral, and Antifungal Activity of Curcumin."

14. Moghadamtousi et al., "A Review of Antibacterial, Antiviral, and Antifungal Activity of Curcumin."

15. Fatemeh Zahedipour et al., "Potential Effects of Curcumin in the Treatment of Covid-19 Infection," *Phytotherapy Research* (May 2020).

16. J. Steinmann et al., "Anti-Infective Properties of Epigallocatechin-3-Gallate (EGCG), a Component of Green Tea," *British Journal of Pharmacology* 168, no. 5 (March 2013): 1059–73.

17. Alexandra Mankovskaia et al., "Catechin-Incorporated Dental Copolymers Inhibit Growth of *Streptococcus mutans*," *Journal of Applied Oral Science* 21, no. 2 (March–April 2013): 203–7.

18. Steinmann et al., "Anti-Infective Properties of Epigallocatechin-3-Gallate (EGCG), a Component of Green Tea."

19. Steinmann et al., "Anti-Infective Properties of Epigallocatechin-3-Gallate (EGCG), a Component of Green Tea."

20. Qiuju Mou et al., "EGCG Induces B-defensin 3 Against Influenza A virus H1N1 by the MAPK Signaling Pathway," *Experimental and Therapeutic Medicine* 20, no. 4 (October 2021): 3017–24.

21. "EGCG (Epigallocatechin Gallate): Benefits, Dosage, and Safety," Healthline website, accessed December 10, 2021.

22. Corey Whelan, "Glutathione Benefits," Healthline website, accessed December 26, 2021.

23. W. Droge and R. Breitkreutz, "Glutathione and Immune Function," *Proceedings of the Nutrition Society* 59, no. 4 (November 2000): 595–600.

24. Roaa Alharbe et al., "Antibacterial Activity of Exogenous Glutathione and Its Synergism on Antibiotics Sensitize Carbapenem-Associated Multidrug-Resistant Clinical Isolates of *Acinetobacter baumanni*," *International Journal of Medical Microbiology* 307, no. 7 (October 2017): 409–14.

25. Aoife Howard et al., *"Acinetobacter baumannii,"* *Virulence* 3, no. 3 (May 1, 2012): 243–50.

26. YaNi Zhang and KangMin Duan, "Glutathione Exhibits Antibacterial Activity and Increases Tetracycline Efficacy Against *Pseudomonas aeruginosa*," *Science in China, Series C, Life Sciences* 52, no. 6 (June 2009): 501–5.

27. Alexey Polonikov, "Endogenous Deficiency of Glutathione as the Most Likely Cause of Serious Manifestations and Death in Covid-19 Patients," *ACS Infectious Diseases* 6, no. 7 (May 28, 2020): 1558–62.

28. A. Khanfar and B. Al Qaroot, "Could Glutathione Depletion Be the Trojan Horse of Covid-19 Mortality?" *European Review for Medical and Pharmacological Sciences* 24, no. 23 (December 2020): 12500–09.

29. David C. Fajgenbaum, and Carl H. June, "Cytokine Storms," *New England Journal of Medicine* 383 (December 3, 2020): 2255–73.

30. Carlo Perriconne et al., "Glutathione: A Key Player in Autoimmunity," *Autoimmunity Reviews* 8, no. 8 (July 2009): 697–701.

31. Whelan, "Glutathione Benefits."

32. Whelan, "Glutathione Benefits."

33. Chandrika J. Piyathilake et al., "Indian Women with Higher Serum Concentrations of Folate and Vitamin B12 Are Significantly Less Likely to be Infected with Carcinogenic or High-Risk (HR) Types of Human Papillomaviruses (HPVs)," *International Journal of Women's Health* 2 (August 9, 2010): 7–12.

34. Kristy Minton, "Magnesium Regulates Antiviral Immunity," *Nature Reviews: Immunology* 13 (July 19, 2013): 548–49.

35. Anne Marie Uwitonze and Mohammed S. Razzaque, "Role of Magnesium in Vitamin D Activation and Function," *Journal of the American Osteopathic Association* 118, no. 3 (March 1, 2018): 181–89.

36. James J. DiNicolantonio et al., "Subclinical Magnesium Deficiency: A Principal Driver of Cardiovascular Disease and a Public Health Crisis," *Open Heart* 5, no. 1 (2018).

37. Mohammed S. Razzaque, "Magnesium: Are We Consuming Enough?" *Nutrients* 10 no. 12 (December 2, 2018): 1863.

38. DiNicolantonio et al., "Subclinical Magnesium Deficiency: A Principal Driver of Cardiovascular Disease and a Public Health Crisis."

39. Eduardo P. Amaral et al., "N-Acetyl-Cystein Exhibits Potent Anti-Mycobacterial Activity in Addition to its Known Anti-Oxidative Functions," *BMC Microbiology* 16, no. 1 (October 28, 2016): 251.

40. N. Rastogi et al., "The Mycobacteria: An Introduction to Nomenclature and Pathogenesis," *Revue Scientifique et Technique* 20, no. 1 (April 2001): 21–54.

41. Amaral et al., "N-Acetyl-Cystein Exhibits Potent Anti-Mycobacterial Activity in Addition to its Known Anti-Oxidative Functions," 251.

42. S. Dinicola et al, "N-Acetyl Cysteine as Powerful Molecule to Destroy Bacterial Biofilms: A Systematic Review," *European Review for Medical and Pharmacological Sciences* 18, no. 19 (October 2014): 2942–48.

43. Ruoqiong Cao et al., "Characterizing the Effects of Glutathione as an Immunoadjuvant in the Treatment of Tuberculosis," *Antimicrobial Agents and Chemotherapy* 62, no. 11 (October 24, 2018): e01132–18.

44. Vida Mokhtari et al, "A Review on Various Uses of N-Acetyl Cysteine," *Cell Journal* 19, no. 1 (April–June 2017):11–17.

45. Silvio de Flora et al., "Rationale for the Use of N-Acetyl in Both Prevention and Adjuvant Therapy of COVID-19," *FASEB Journal* 34, no. 10 (October 2020): 13185–93.

46. Yao Wang et al., "N-Acetyl Cysteine Effectively Alleviates Coxsackie-B-Induced Myocarditis Through Suppressing Viral Replication and Inflammatory Response," *Antiviral Research* 179 (July 2020): 104699.

47. Philip C. Calder, "Nutrition, Immunity, and Covid-19," *BMJ Nutrition, Prevention, & Health* 3, no. 1 (May 30, 2020): 74–92.

48. "Quercetin: Uses, Side Effects, and More," WebMD, accessed December 13, 2021.

49. Ryan Beesley, "Quercetin—An Alternative to Hydroxychloroquine, and More," Fox News website, accessed December 29, 2021.

50. Ruben Manuel Luciano Colunga Biancatelli et al., "Quercetin and Vitamin C: An Experimental, Synergistic Therapy for the Prevention and Treatment of SARS-CoV-2 Related Disease (Covid-19)," *Frontiers in Immunology* (June 19, 2020).

51. Wenjiao Wu et al., "Quercetin as an Antiviral Agent Inhibits Influenza A Virus (IAV) Entry," *Viruses* 8, no. 1 (December 24, 2015): 6.

52. Charles Patrick David, "Medical Definition of RNA Virus," MedicineNet website, accessed December 13, 2021.

53. Biancatelli et al., "Quercetin and Vitamin C."

54. Biancatelli et al., "Quercetin and Vitamin C."

55. Calder, "Nutrition, Immunity, and Covid-19."

56. Laurent Hiffler and Benjamin Rakotoambinina, "Selenium and RNA Virus Interactions: Potential Implications for SARS-CoV-2 Infection (COVID-19)," *Frontiers in Nutrition* 7 (September 4, 2020): 164.

57. David, "Medical Definition of RNA Virus."

58. Jan Alexander et al., "Early Nutritional Interventions with Zinc, Selenium, and Vitamin D for Raising Anti-Viral Resistance Against Progressive Covid-19," *Nutrients* 12, no. 8 (August 7, 2020): 2358.

59. Natalie Olsen, "20 Foods Rich in Selenium," Healthline website, accessed December 30, 2021.

60. Colunga Biancatelli, M. Berrill, and P. E. Marik. "The Antiviral Properties of Vitamin C." *Expert Review of Anti-Infective Therapy* 18 (2020): 99–101.

61. Biancatelli et al., "Quercetin and Vitamin C."

62. Biancatelli et al., "Quercetin and Vitamin C."

63. Biancatelli et al., "Quercetin and Vitamin C."

64. Zhila Maghbooli et al., "Vitamin D Deficiency, a Serum 25-Hydroxyvitamin D at Least 30 ng/mL Reduced Risk for Adverse Clinical Outcomes in Patients with Covid-19 Infection," *PLOS One* (September 25, 2020).

65. Somaieh Matin et al., "The Sufficient Vitamin D and Albumin Level Have a Protective Effect on COVID-19 Infection," *Archives of Microbiology* 203 (July 30, 2021): 5153–62.

66. Francesca Sassi et al., "Vitamin D: Nutrient, Hormone, and Immunomodulator," *Nutrients* 10, no. 11 (November 3, 2018): 1656.

67. Sassi et al., "Vitamin D."

68. Sizar et al., "Vitamin D Deficiency," *StatPearls* (July 21, 2020), accessed December 9, 2021.

69. Miriam A. Guevara et al., "Vitamin D and *Streptococci:* The Interface of Nutrition, Host Immune Response, and Antimicrobial Activity, in Response to Infection," *ACS Infectious Diseases* 6, no. 12 (December 11, 2020): 3131–40.

70. Maghbooli et al., "Vitamin D Deficiency."

71. Joseph Mercola et al., "Evidence Regarding Vitamin D and Risk of COVID-19 and Its Severity," *Nutrients* 12, no. 11 (October 31, 2020): 3361.

72. Gaelle Annweiler et al., "Vitamin D Supplementation Associated to Better Survival in Hospitalized Frail Elderly COVID-19 Patients: The GERIA-COVID Quasi-Experimental Study," *Nutrients* 12, no. 11 (November 2, 2020): 3377.

73. Mercola et al., "Evidence Regarding Vitamin D and Risk of COVID-19 and Its Severity."

74. Annweiler et al., "Vitamin D Supplementation Associated to Better Survival in Hospitalized Frail Elderly COVID-19 Patients."

75. Sizar et al., "Vitamin D Deficiency."

76. Sizar et al., "Vitamin D Deficiency."

77. Bo Li et al., "Zinc Regulation System in Bacteria and Its Relationship with Infection—A Review," *Acta Microbiologica Sinica* 56, no. 8 (August 4, 2016): 1211–21.

78. Qian Ye et al., "Iron and Zinc Ions, Potent Weapons Against Multidrug-Resistant Bacteria," *Applied Microbiology and Biotechnology* 104, no. 12 (June 2020): 5213–27.

79. Ahmet Sami Yazar et al., "Effects of Zinc or Synbiotic on the Duration of Diarrhea in Children with Acute Infectious Diarrhea," *Turkish Journal of Gastroenterology* 27, no. 6 (November 2016): 537–40.

80. Jun Xie et al., "Zinc Supplementation Reduces *Candida* Infections in Pediatric Intensive Care Unit: A Randomized-, Placebo-Controlled Clinical Trial," *Journal of Clinical Biochemistry and Nutrition* 64, no. 2 (March 2019): 170–73.

81. Scott Read et al., "The Role of Zinc in Antiviral Immunity," *Advances in Nutrition* 10, no. 4 (July 1, 2019): 696–710.

82. "Zinc," Mayo Clinic website, accessed December 27, 2021.

83. Inga Wessels et al., "The Potential Impact of Zinc Supplementation on Covid-19 Pathogenesis," *Frontiers in Immunology* 11 (July 10, 2020): 1712.

84. Read et al., "The Role of Zinc in Antiviral Immunity," 696–k710.

85. "Zinc," Mayo Clinic website, accessed December 27, 2021.

86. "Vitamins and Minerals: How Much Should You Take?" WebMD, accessed December 9, 2021.

87. "Berberine: Uses, Side Effects, and More," WebMD, accessed December 9, 2021.

88. "Turmeric: Uses, Side Effects, and More," WebMD, accessed December 9, 2021.

89. Jiang Hu et al., "The Safety of Green Tea and Green Tea Extract Consumption in Adults—Results of a Systematic Review," *Regulatory Toxicology and Pharmacology* 95 (June 2018): 412–33.

90. R. Morgan Griffin, "Folate (Folic Acid," WebMD, accessed October 18, 2022.

91. R. Morgan Griffin, "Magnesium," WebMD, accessed October 18, 2022.

92. "N-acetyl Cysteine (Nac): Uses, Side Effects, and More," WebMD, accessed December 9, 2021.

93. "Quercetin: Uses, Side Effects, and More," WebMD, accessed December 13, 2021.

94. Jillian Levy, "Selenium Benefits, Foods, Dosage and Side Effects," Dr. Axe website, April 3, 2022, accessed October 18, 2022.

95. Omudhome Ogbru, "Oral Cyanocobalamin (Vitamin B-12)," Medicinenet, accessed October 18, 2022.

96. Ba X. Hoang et al., "Possible Application of High-Dose Vitamin C in the Prevention and Therapy of Coronavirus Infection," *Journal of Global Antimicrobial Resistance* 23 (December 2020): 256–62.

97. Ryan Raman, "What Vitamin D Dosage Is Best?" Healthline website, October 8, 2017, accessed October 18, 2022.

98. Read et al., "The Role of Zinc in Antiviral Immunity."

99. Calder, "Nutrition, Immunity, and Covid-19," 74–92.

100. Rachel Link, "15 Healthy Foods That Are High in Folate (Folic Acid)," Healthline website, accessed December 30, 2021.

101. Calder, "Nutrition, Immunity, and Covid-19," 74–92.

102. Helen West, RD, "8 Foods That Are High in Copper," Healthline website, accessed December 30, 2021.

103. Calder, "Nutrition, Immunity, and Covid-19," 74–92.

104. Zhiyi Huang et al., "Role of Vitamin A in the Immune System," *Journal of Clinical Medicine* 7, no. 9 (2018), 258.

105. Vaughn S. Somerville et al., "Effect of Flavonoids on Upper Respiratory Tract Infections and Immune Function: A Systematic Review and Meta-Analysis," *Advances in Nutrition* 7, no. 3 (May 2016): 488–97.

106. Analy Machado de Oliveira Leite et al., "Microbiological, Technological, and Therapeutic Properties of Kefir: A Natural Probiotic Beverage," *Brazilian Journal of Microbiology* 44, no. 2 (October 30, 2013): 341–49.

107. Kun-Young Park et al., "Health Benefits of Kimchi (Korean Fermented Vegetables) as a Probiotic Food," *Journal of Medicinal Food* 17, no. 1 (January 2014): 6–20.

108. K. Watanabe et al., "Anti-Influenza Viral Effects of Honey in Vitro: Potent High Activity of Manuka Honey," *Archives of Medical Research* 45, no. 5 (July 2014): 359–65.

CHAPTER 3. HERBS AND ESSENTIAL OILS

1. J. da Silva et al., "Essential Oils as Antiviral Agents, Potential of Essential Oils to Treat SARS-Cov-2 Infection: An In Silico Investigation," *International Journal of Molecular Sciences* 21, no. 10 (May 2020): 3426.

2. A. Astani et al., "Comparative Study on the Antiviral Activity of Selected Monoterpenes Derived from Essential Oils," *Phytotherapy Research* 24, no. 5 (May 2010): 673–79.

3. "Cold Versus Flu," Centers for Disease Control and Prevention website, accessed May 10, 2021.

4. Valentina Virginia Ebani et al., "Antimicrobial Activity of Five Essential Oils Against Bacteria and Fungi Responsible for Urinary Tract infections," *Molecules* 23, no. 7 (July 9, 2018): 1668.

5. Abdella Gemechu et al., "In Vitro Anti-Mycobacterial Activity of Selected Medicinal Plants Against *Mycobacterium tuberculosis* and *Mycobacterium bovis* Strains," *BMC Complementary and Alternative Medicine* 13 (October 29, 2013): 291.

6. Danilo Alfaro, "What Is Cumin?" The Spruce Eats website, accessed January 10, 2022.

7. Qing Liu et al., "Antibacterial and Antifungal Activity of Spices," *International Journal of Molecular Sciences* 18, no. 6 (June 16, 2017): 1283.

8. Naina Mohamed Pakkir Maideen, "Prophetic Medicine—Nigella sativa (Black Cumin Seeds)—Potential Herb for Covid-19?" *Journal of Pharmacopuncture* 23, no. 2 (June 30, 2020): 62–70.

9. Maideen, "Prophetic Medicine—Nigella sativa (Black Cumin Seeds)—Potential Herb for Covid-19?" 62–70.

10. Maideen, "Prophetic Medicine—Nigella sativa (Black Cumin Seeds)—Potential Herb for Covid-19?" 62–70.

11. Abdul Hannan et al., "Antibacterial Activity of *Nigella sativa* Against Clinical Isolates of Methicillin-Resistant *Staphylococcus aureus*," *Journal of Ayub Medical College* 20, no. 3 (July–September 2008): 72–74.

12. Josh Axe, "9 Proven Black Seed Oil Benefits That Boost Your Health," Dr. Axe website, February 10, 2020.

13. Mohd Tariq Salman, "Antimicrobial Activity of *Nigella sativa Linn.* Seed Oil Against Multi-Drug Resistant Bacteria from Clinical Isolates," *Natural Product Radiance* 7 no. 1 (January 2008).

14. Josh Axe, "9 Proven Black Seed Oil Benefits That Boost Your Health."

15. "List B: EPA's Registered Tuberculocide Products Effective Against *Mycobacterium tuberculosis*," United States Environmental Protection Agency website, accessed January 10, 2022.

16. M. Taha et al., "Antifungal Effect of Thymol, Thymoquinone, and Thymohydroquinone Against Yeasts, Dermatophytes, and Non-Dermatophyte Molds Isolated from Skin and Nails Fungal Infections," *Egyptian Journal of Biochemistry and Molecular Biology* 28, no. 2 (2010).

17. Edgar Garter, "The Cat's Claw: A Miracle Cure from the Jungle," *European Scientist* (April 23, 2018).

18. Daniel Rodrigo Herrera et al., "Antimicrobial Activity and Substantivity of *Uncaria tomentosa* in Infected Root Canal Dentin," *Brazilian Oral Research* 30, no. 1 (2016): e61.

19. Renzo Alberto Ccahuana-Vasquez et al., "Antimicrobial Activity of *Uncaria tomentosa* Against Oral Human Pathogens," *Brazilian Oral Research* 21, no. 1 (January–March 2007): 46–50.

20. Garter, "The Cat's Claw."

21. Thiago Caon et al., "Antimutagenic and Antiherpetic Activities of Different Preparations from *Uncaria tomentosa* (Cat's Claw)," *Food and Chemical Toxicology* 66 (April 2014): 30–35.

22. Andres F. Yepes-Perez et al. "*Uncaria tomentosa* (Cat's Claw): A Promising Herbal Medicine Against SARS-CoV-2/ACE-2 Junction and SARS-CoV-2

Spike Protein Based on Molecular Modeling," *Journal of Biomolecular Structure and Dynamics* (October 29, 2020): 1–17.

23. Garter, "The Cat's Claw."

24. Garter, "The Cat's Claw."

25. Mohamed A. Jollah et al., "Dietary Supplement Interactions with Antiretrovirals: A Systematic Review," *International Journal of STD & AIDS* 28, no. 1 (January 2017): 4–15.

26. Mary Jane Brown, "Cat's Claw: Benefits, Side Effects, and Dosage," Healthline website, accessed February 9, 2022.

27. "Topic Overview: What Is Chamomile?" WebMD, accessed January 3, 2022.

28. H. Rahman and A. Chandra, "Microbiologic Evaluation of Matricaria and Chlorhexadine Against *E. faecalis* and *C. albicans,*" *Indian Journal of Dentistry* 6, no. 2 (2015): 60–64.

29. Christine Koch, et al., "Efficacy of Anise Oil, Dwarf-Pine Oil, and Chamomile Oil Against Thymidine-Kinase-Positive and Thymidine-Kinase-Negative Herpesviruses," *Journal of Pharmacy and Pharmacology* 60, no. 11 (November 2008): 1545–50.

30. Joe Leech, "Ceylon vs. Cassia: Not All Cinnamon Is Created Equal," Healthline website, accessed November 30, 2021.

31. N. D. Vasconcelos et al., "Antibacterial Mechanisms of Cinnamon and Its Constituents: A Review," *Microbial Pathogenesis* 120 (July 2018): 198–203.

32. Rasheeha Naveed et al., "Antimicrobial Activity of the Bioactive Components of Essential Oils from Pakistani Species Against Salmonella and Other Multi-Drug Resistant Bacteria," *BMC Complementary and Alternative Medicine* 13 (October 14, 2013): 265.

33. Kamilla Acs et al., "Antibacterial Activity Evaluation of Selected Essential Oils in Liquid and Vapor Phase on Respiratory Tract Pathogens," *BMC Complementary and Alternative Medicines* 18, no. 1 (July 27, 2018): 227.

34. Spartak Yanakiev, "Effects of Cinnamon (*Cinnamomum spp.*) in Dentistry: A Review," *Molecules* 25, no. 18 (September 12, 2020): 4184.

35. A. Brochot et al. "Antibacterial, Antifungal, and Antiviral Effects of Three Essential Oil Blends," *Microbiology Open* 6, no. 4 (August 6, 2017).

36. M. Fatima et al., "In Vitro Antiviral Activity of *Cinnamomum cassia* and Its Nanoparticles Against H7N3 Influenza A Virus," *Journal of Microbiology and Biotechnology* 26, no. 1 (January 2016): 151–59.

37. Kurt Schnaubelt, *Advanced Aromatherapy: The Science of Essential Oil Therapy* (Rochester, Vt.: Healing Arts Press, 1995), 65.

38. Elgio Venanda Ginting et al., "Antibacterial Activity of Clove (*Szygium aromaticum*) and Cinnamon (*Cinnamomum burmannii*) Essential Oil Against Extended-Spectrum B-Lactamase-Producing Bacteria," *Veterinary World* 14, no. 8 (August 2021): 2206–11.

39. Kamel Chaieb et al., "Antioxidant Properties of the Essential Oil of *Eugenia caryophyllata* and Its Antifungal Activity Against a Large Number of Clinical *Candida* Species," *Mycoses* 50, no. 5 (September 2007): 403–6.

40. Thomas Lane et al., "The Natural Product Eugenol Is an Inhibitor of the Ebola Virus in Vitro," *Pharmaceutical Research* 36, no. 7 (May 17, 2019): 104.

41. Kamel Chaieb et al, "The Chemical Composition and Biological Activity of Clove Essential Oil, *Eugenia caryophyllata* (*Syzigium aromaticum L. Myrtacea*): A Short Review," *Phytotherapy Research* (March 23, 2007).

42. Y. Tragoolpua and A. Jatisatienr, "Anti-Herpes Simplex Virus Activities of *Eugenia Caryophyllus* (Spreng.) and Essential Oil, Eugenol," *Phytotherapy Research* 21, no. 12 (December 2007): 1153–58.

43. Ryan Raman, "Echinacea: Benefits, Uses, Side Effects and Dosage," Healthline website, October 25, 2018.

44. David Hoffman, *Medical Herbalism: The Science and Practice of Herbal Medicine* (Rochester, Vt.: Healing Arts Press, 2003), 544.

45. A. Schapowal et al., "Echinacea Reduces the Risk of Recurrent Respiratory Tract Infections and Complications: A Meta-Analysis of Randomized Controlled Trials," *Advances in Therapy* 32, no. 3 (March 2015): 187–200.

46. D. J. Fast et al., "*Echinacea purpurea* Root Extract Inhibits TNF Release I Response to Pam3Csk4 in a Phosphatidylinositol-3 Kinase-Dependent Manner," *Cell Immunology* 297, no. 2 (July 2015): 94–99.

47. Joanna Signer et al., "In Vitro Virucidal Activity of Echinaforce, an *Echinacea purpurea* Preparation Against Coronaviruses, Including Common Cold Coronavirus 229E and SARS-CoV-2," *Virology Journal* (September 9, 2020).

48. B. Barrett, "Medicinal Properties of Echinacea: A Critical Review," *Phytomedicine* 1 (January 2003): 66–86.

49. D. Charlebois, "Elderberry as a Medicinal Plant," *Issues in New Crops and New Uses* (Alexandria, Va.: ASHS Press, 2007).

50. Emiko Kinoshita et al., "Anti-Influenza Virus Effects of Elderberry Juice and Its Fractions," *Bioscience, Biotechnology, and Biochemistry* 76, no. 9 (2012): 1633–38.

51. Jing-Ru Weng et al., "Antiviral Activity of *Sambuca formosanaNakai* Ethanol Extract and Related Phenolic Acid Constituents Against Human Coronavirus NL63," *Virus Research* 273 (November 2019): 197767.

52. Xin Li et al., "Human Coronaviruses: General Features," *Reference Module in Biomedical Sciences* (2019).

53. Hoffman, *Medical Herbalism,* 580.

54. Jessie Hawkins et al., "Black Elderberry (*Sambucus nigra*) Supplementation Effectively Treats Upper Respiratory Symptoms: A Meta-Analysis of Randomized, Controlled Clinical Trials," *Complementary Therapies in Medicine* 42 (February 2019): 361–65.

55. V. Barak et al., "The Effect of Sambucol, a Black Elderberry-Based Natural Product, on the Production of Human Cytokines: I. Inflammatory Cytokines," *European Cytokine Network* 12, no. 2 (April–June 2001): 20–6.

56. Tatiana V. Kirichenko et al., "Anti-Cytokine Therapy for Prevention of Atherosclerosis," *Phytomedicine* 23, no. 11 (October 15, 2016): 1198–210.

57. C. N. Tiboc Schnell et al., "The Impact of *Sambucus nigra L.* Extract on Inflammation, Oxidative Stress, and Tissue Remodeling in a Rat Model of Lipopolysaccharide-Induced Subacute Rhinosinusitis," *Inflammopharmacology* 29, no. 3 (June 2021): 753–69.

58. M. Castelman, *The New Healing Herbs* (New York: Bantam Books, 2003), 286.

59. Castelman, *The New Healing Herbs,* 287.

60. J. A. Duke, *The Green Pharmacy* (Emmaus, Penn.: Rodale Press, 1997), 297.

61. Duke, *The Green Pharmacy,* 166.

62. S. Ankri and D. Mirelman, "Antimicrobial Properties of Allicin in Garlic," *Microbes and Infection* 1, no. 2 (February 1999): 125–29.

63. Razina Rouf et al., "Antiviral Potential of Garlic (*Allium sativum*) and Its Organosulfur Compounds: A Systematic Update of Pre-Clinical and Clinical Data," *Trends in Food Science and Technology* 104 (October 2020): 219–34.

64. Hoffman, *Medical Herbalism,* 526.

65. K. Priebe, "Know Your Spice: A Brief History of Ginger," *Mother Earth Living* (March 16, 2011).

66. Stephen Harrod Buhner, *Herbal Antivirals: Natural Remedies for Emerging and Resistant Viral Infections* (North Adams, Mass.: Storey Publishing, 2013).

67. Agnes Peterfalvi et al., "Much More Than a Pleasant Scent: A Review of Essential Oils Supporting the Immune System," *Molecules* (December 11, 2019).

68. Jung San Chang et al., "Fresh Ginger (*Zingiber officinale*) has Anti-Viral Activity Against Human Respiratory Syncytial Virus in Human Respiratory Tract Cell Lines," *Journal of Ethnopharmacology* 145, no. 1 (January 9, 2013): 146–51.

69. Amir Rasool, et al., "Anti-avian Influenza Virus (H9N2) Activity of Aqueous Extracts of Zingiber officinalis (Ginger) and Allium sativum (Garlic) in Chick Embryos," *Pakistan Journal of Pharmaceutical Sciences* 30, no. 4 (July 2017); 1341–44.

70. Hoffman, *Medical Herbalism,* 597.

71. Hoffman, *Medical Herbalism,* 566.

72. Fahima Abdellatif et al., "Minerals, Essential Oils, and Biological Properties of *Melissa officinalis* L.," *Plants* 10, no. 6 (May 26, 2021): 1066.

73. Elisa Serra et al., "Methylcellulose Hydrogel with *Melissa officinalis* Essential Oil as a Potential Treatment for Oral Candidiasis," *Microorganisms* 8, no. 2 (February 6, 2020): 215.

74. "Oral Thrush," Mayo Clinic website, accessed February 15, 2022.

75. Akram Astani et al., "*Melissa officinalis* Extract Inhibits Attachment of Herpes Simplex Virus in Vitro," *Chemotherapy* 58, no. 1 (2012): 70–77.

76. Hoffman, *Medical Herbalism,* 566.

77. G. Mazzanti et al., "Inhibitory Activity of *Melissa officinalis L.* Extract on *Herpes Simplex* Virus Type 2 Replication," *Natural Product Research* 22, no. 16 (2008): 1433–40.

78. S. Geuenich et al., "Aqueous Extract from Peppermint, Sage, and Lemon Balm Leaves Display Potent Anti-HIV-1 Activity by Increasing the Virion Density," *Retrovirology* 5 (March 20, 2008): 27.

79. D. Winston and S. Maimes, *Adaptogens: Herbs for Strength, Stamina, and Stress Relief* (Rochester, Vt.: Healing Arts Press, 2007), 175.

80. Winston and Maimes, *Adaptogens,* 171.

81. Liqiang Wang et al., "The Antiviral and Antimicrobial Activities of Licorice, a Widely-Used Chinese Herb," *Acta Pharmaceutica Sinica B* 5, no. 4 (2015): 310–15.

82. M. Lee et al., "Quercetin-Induced Apoptosis Prevents EPV Infection," *Oncotarget* 6, no. 14 (May 2015): 12603–24.

83. Hoffman, *Medical Herbalism,* 554–55.

84. A. Wani et al., "An Updated and Comprehensive Review of the Antiviral Potential of Essential Oils and Their Chemical Constituents with Special Focus on their Mechanism of Action Against Various Influenza and Coronaviruses," *Microbial Pathogenesis* 152 (March 2021).

85. Christine Ruggeri, "Olive Leaf Extract Benefits Cardiovascular Health and Brain Function," Dr. Axe website, June 12, 2019.

86. D. Markin et al., "In Vitro Antimicrobial Activity of Olive Leaves," *Mycoses* 46, no. 3–4 (April 2003): 132–36.

87. Ruggeri, "Olive Leaf Extract Benefits Cardiovascular Health and Brain Function."

88. Ruggeri, "Olive Leaf Extract Benefits Cardiovascular Health and Brain Function."

89. Sylvia Lee-Huang et al., "Anti-HIV Activity of Olive Leaf Extract (OLE) and Modulation of Host Cell Gene Expression by HIV-1 Infection and OLE Treatment," *Biochemical and Biophysical Research Communications* 307, no. 4 (August 8, 2003): 1029–37.

90. Ruggeri, "Olive Leaf Extract Benefits Cardiovascular Health and Brain Function."

91. Kerry Kolasa-Sikiaridi, "Oregano: The Quintessential Ancient Greek Herb," *Greek Reporter* (March 10, 2022).

92. G. Magi et al., "Antimicrobial Activity of Essential Oils and Carvacrol, and Synergy of Carvacrol and Erythromycin, Against Clinical Erythromycin-Resistant, Group A Streptococci," *Frontiers in Microbiology* 6 (March 3, 2015): 165.

93. M. Fournomiti et al., "Antimicrobial Activity of Essential Oils of Cultivated Oregano (*Origanum vulgare*), Sage (*Salvia officinalis*), and Thyme (*Thymus vulgaris*) against Clinical Isolates of *Escherichia coli*, *Klebsiella oxytoca*, and *Klebsielle pneumoniae*," *Microbial Ecology in Health and Disease* 26 (April 15, 2015): 23289.

94. Magi et al., "Antimicrobial Activity of Essential Oils and Carvacrol, and Synergy of Carvacrol and Erythromycin, Against Clinical Erythromycin-Resistant Group A Streptococci."

95. S. Mediouni et al., "Oregano Oil and Its Principal Component, Carvacrol, Inhibit HIV-1 Fusion into Cells," *Journal of Virology* 94, no. 15 (August 2020).

96. S. Mediouni et al., "Oregano Oil and Its Principal Component, Carvacrol, Inhibit HIV-1 Fusion into Target Cells," *Journal of Virology* 94, no. 15 (July 16, 2020): e00147–20.

97. "Peppermint," World's Healthiest Foods website, accessed February 16, 2022.

98. J. Heinerman, *Healing Herbs and Spices* (New York: Reward Books, 1996), 333.

99. Christine Koch et al. "Efficacy of Anise Oil, Dwarf-Pine Oil, and Chamomile Oil Against Thymidine-Kinase-Positive and Thymidine-Kinase-Negative Herpes Viruses," *Journal of Pharmacy and Pharmacology* 60, no. 11 (November 2008): 1545–50.

100. Athbi Alqareer et al., "The Effect of Clove and Benzocaine Versus Placebo as Topical Anesthetics," *Journal of Dentistry* 34, no. 10 (November 2006): 747–50.

101. Akram Astani et al., "Attachment and Penetration of Acyclovir-Resistant Herpes Simplex Virus Are Inhibited by *Melissa officinalis* extract," *Phytotherapy Research* 28, no. 10 (October 2014): 1547–52.

102. Xiao-Li Zhang et al., "Phenolic Compounds from *Origanum vulgare* and Their Antioxidant and Antiviral Activities," *Food Chemistry* 154 (June 2014): 300–306.

103. A. Schumacher et al., "Virucidal Effect of Peppermint Oil on the Enveloped Viruses Herpes Simplex Virus Type 1 and Type 2 in Vitro," *Phytomedicine* 10, no. 6–7 (2003): 504–10.

104. A. Garozzo et al., "In Vitro Antiviral Activity of *Melaleuca alternifolia* Essential Oil," *Letters in Applied Microbiology* 49, no. 6 (December 2009): 806–8.

105. Hoffman, *Medical Herbalism,* 545.

106. Hoffman, *Medical Herbalism,* 545.

107. Jayanta Kumar Patra et al., "Star Anise (*Illicium verum*): Chemical Compounds, Antiviral Properties, and Clinical Relevance," *Phytotherapy Research* 34, no. 6 (June 2020): 1248–67.

108. Tahir Mahmood Khan, "Use of Star Anise Tea in Swine Flue [*sic*] Prevention and Safety Concerns," *Complementary Therapies in Clinical Practice* 16, no. 3, (August 2010): 175.

109. Magi et al., "Antimicrobial Activity of Essential Oils and Carvacrol and Synergy of Carvacrol and Erythromycin Against Clinical Erythromycin-Resistant Group A Streptococci," 165.

110. X. Li et al., "*Melaleuca alternifolia* Concentrate Inhibits In Vitro Entry of Influenza Virus into Host Cells," *Molecules* 18, no. 8 (August 9, 2019): 9550–66.

111. Hercules Sakkas and Chrissanthy Papadopoulou, "Antimicrobial Activity of Basil, Oregano and Thyme Essential Oils," *Journal of Microbiology and Biotechnology* 27, no. 3 (2017): 429–38.

112. Valentina Virginia Ebani et al., "Antimicrobial Activity of Five Essential Oils Against Bacteria and Fungi Responsible for Urinary Tract Infections," *Molecules* 23, no. 7 (July 9, 2018): 1668.

113. Kamilla Acs et al., "Antibacterial Activity Evaluation of Selected Essential Oils in Liquid and Vapor Phase on Respiratory Tract Pathogens," *BMC Complementary and Alternative Medicine* 18, no. 1 (July 27, 2018): 227.

114. Mohd S. A. Khan et al., "*Carum coptum* and *Thymus vulgaris* Oils Inhibit Virulence in *Trichophytum rubrum* and *Aspergillus* spp.," *Brazilian Journal of Microbiology* 45, no. 2 (August 29, 2014): 523–31.

115. Mohd S. A. Khan et al., "Sub-MICs of *Carum capticum* and *Thymus vulgaris* Influence Virulence Factors and Biofilm Formation in *Candida* spp.," *BMC Complementary and Alternative Medicine* 14 (September 15, 2014): 337.

116. A. Astani et al., "Comparative Study on the Antiviral Activity of Selected Monoterpenes Derived from Essential Oils," *Phytotherapy Research* 24, no. 5 (May 2010): 673–79.

117. Duke, *The Green Pharmacy,* 289.

118. Jie Feng et al., "Identification of Essential Oils with Strong Activity against Stationary Phase *Borrelia burgdorferi,*" *Antibiotics* 7, no. 4 (October 16, 2018).

119. Ana Sandoiu, "These 10 Essential Oils Can Kill Persistent Lyme Disease," Medical News Today website, December 4, 2018.

120. Marjorie Hecht, "13 Signs and Symptoms of Lyme Disease," Healthline website, accessed February 22, 2022.

121. Jie Feng et al., "Selective Essential Oils from Spice or Culinary Herbs Have High Activity Against Stationary Phase and Biofilm *Borrelia burgdorferi,*" *Frontiers in Medicine* 4 (2017): 169.

CHAPTER 4. PROBIOTICS AND FERMENTED FOODS

1. G. Vighi et al., "Allergy and the Gastrointestinal System," *Clinical and Experimental Immunology* 153, no. 1 (September 2008): 3–6.

2. Erika C. Claud and W. Allen Walker, "The Intestinal Microbiota and the

Microbiome," *Gastroenterology and Nutrition: Neonatal Questions and Controversies* (2008).

3. Mary Ellen Sanders, "Probiotics: Definition, Selection, Sources, and Uses," *Clinical Infectious Diseases* 46, no. S2 (2008): S58–61.

4. Donatella Comito, Antonio Cascio, and Claudio Romano, "Microbiota Biodiversity in Inflammatory Bowel Disease," *Italian Journal of Pediatrics* (March 31, 2014).

5. Philip C. Calder, "Nutrition, Immunity, and Covid-19," *BMJ Nutrition, Prevention, & Health* 3, no. 1 (May 30, 2020): 74–92.

6. Mary Ellen Sanders, "How Do We Know When Something Called 'Probiotic' Is Really a Probiotic? A Guideline for Consumers and Health Care Professionals," *Functional Food Reviews* 1, no. 1 (Spring 2009): 3–12.

7. Lucia Pacifico et al. "Probiotics for the Treatment of *Helicobacter pylori* Infection in Children," *World Journal of Gastroenterology* (January 21, 201): 673–83.

8. A. Lyra et al. "Comparison of Bacterial Quantities in Left and Right Colon Biopsies and Faeces," *World Journal of Gastroenterology* 18, no. 32 (August 28, 2012): 1404–11.

9. Hempel et al. "Probiotics for the Prevention and Treatment of Antibiotic-Associated Diarrhea: A Systematic Review and Meta-Analysis," *Journal of the American Medical Association* (May 9, 2012).

10. E. Lonnermark et al. "Intake of *Lactobacillus plantarum* Reduces Certain Gastrointestinal Symptoms during Treatment with Antibiotics," *Journal of Clinical Gastroenterology* 44, no. 2 (February 2010): 106–12.

11. M. Popova et al., "Beneficial Effects of Probiotics in Upper Respiratory Tract Infections and Their Mechanical Actions to Antagonize Pathogens," *Journal of Applied Microbiology* 113, no. 6 (July 2012): 1305–18.

12. Popova et al., "Beneficial Effects of Probiotics in Upper Respiratory Tract Infections and Their Mechanical Actions to Antagonize Pathogens."

13. S. Khani et al., "In Vitro Study of the Effect of a Probiotic Bacterium *Lactobacillus rhamnosus* against Herpes Simplex Virus Type 1," *Brazilian Journal of Infectious Diseases* 16, no. 2 (March–April 2012): 129–35.

14. C. Rask et al. "Differential Effect on Cell-Mediated Immunity in Human Volunteers after Intake of Different Lactobacilli," *Clinical Experimental Immunology* 172, no. 2 (May 2013): 321–32.

15. E. Guillemard et al., "Consumption of a Fermented Dairy Product Containing the Probiotic *Lactobacillus casei* DN-114001 Reduces the Duration of Respiratory Infections in the Elderly in a Randomised Controlled Trial," *British Journal of Nutrition* 103, no. 1 (January 2010): 58–68.

16. Anna Berggren et al., "Randomised, Double-Blind, and Placebo-Controlled Study using New Probiotic Lactobacilli for Strengthening the Body Immune Defence Against Viral Infections," *European Journal of Nutrition* 50, no. 3 (April 2011): 203–10.

17. Popova et al. "Beneficial Effects of Probiotics in Upper Respiratory Tract Infections and their Mechanical Actions to Antagonize Pathogens," 1305–18.

18. P. Mastromarino et al. "Antiviral Activity of *Lactobacillus brevis* towards Herpes Simplex Virus Type 2: Role of Cell Wall Associated Components," *Anaerobe* 17, no. 6 (December 2011): 334–36.

19. E. I. Ermolenko, "Inhibition of Herpes Simplex Virus Type 1 Reproduction by Probiotic Bacteria in Vitro," *Voprosy Virusologii* 55, no. 4 (July–August 2010): 25–28.

20. T. M. Liaskovs'kyi et al. "Effect of Probiotic Lactic Acid Bacteria Strains on Virus Infection" *Mikrobiolohichnyi zhurnal* 69, no. 2 (March/April 2007): 55–63.

21. H. Hu et al. "Impact of Eating Probiotic Yogurt on Colonization by *Candida* Species of the Oral and Vaginal Mucosa in HIV-Infected and HIV-Uninfected Women," *Mycopathologia* 176, no. 3–4 (October 2013): 175–81.

22. Samuel J. Spaiser et al., "*Lactobacillus gasseri* KS-13, *Bifidobacterium bifidum* G9-1, and *Bifidobacterium longum* MM-2 Ingestion Induces a Less Inflammatory Cytokine Profile and a Potentially Beneficial Shift in Gut Microbiota in Older Adults: A Randomized, Double-Blind, Placebo-Controlled, Crossover Study," *Journal of the American College of Nutrition* 34, no. 6 (2015): 459–69.

CHAPTER 5. MUSHROOMS

1. Karolina Zaremba, "Top 8 Mushrooms for Immune Health," Fullscript blog, September 11, 2020.

2. Luigi Capasso, "5300 Years Ago, the Ice Man Used Natural Laxatives and Antibiotics," *Lancet* 352, no. 9143 (December 5, 1998).

3. Zaremba, "Top 8 Mushrooms for Immune Health."

4. Robert Rogers, *The Fungal Pharmacy: The Complete Guide to Medicinal Mushrooms & Lichens of North America* (Berkeley, Calif.: North Atlantic Books, 2011), 233.

5. Zaremba, "Top 8 Mushrooms for Immune Health."

6. Rogers, *The Fungal Pharmacy,* 235.

7. Rogers, *The Fungal Pharmacy,* 236.

8. Zaremba, "Top 8 Mushrooms for Immune Health."

9. Rogers, *The Fungal Pharmacy,* 121.

10. Zaremba, "Top 8 Mushrooms for Immune Health."

11. Zaremba, "Top 8 Mushrooms for Immune Health."

12. Zaremba, "Top 8 Mushrooms for Immune Health."

13. Rogers, *The Fungal Pharmacy,* 344.

14. Rogers, *The Fungal Pharmacy,* 3443–46.

15. Rogers, *The Fungal Pharmacy,* 172–75.

16. Rogers, *The Fungal Pharmacy,* 175.

17. Xiaoshuang Dai, et al., "Consuming *Lentinula edodes* (Shiitake) Mushrooms Daily Improves Human Immunity: A Randomized, Dietary Intervention in Healthy Young Adults," *Journal of the American College of Nutrition* 34, no. 6 (2015): 478–87.

18. Rogers, *The Fungal Pharmacy,* 400–407.

19. Rogers, *The Fungal Pharmacy,* 410.

20. Rogers, *The Fungal Pharmacy,* 408.

21. Rogers, *The Fungal Pharmacy,* 410.

22. Rogers, *The Fungal Pharmacy,* 503–11.

23. Peter C. B. Turnbull, "Chapter 15: Bacillus," in *Medical Microbiology;* 4th ed., S. Baron, Ed. (Galveston: University of Texas Medical Branch at Galveston, 1996). Available at the National Library of Medicine website, accessed January 21, 2022.

24. "*E. coli,*" Mayo Clinic website, accessed January 21, 2022.

25. Issar Smith, "*Mycobacterium tuberculosis:* Pathogenesis and Molecular Determinants of Virulence," *Clinical Microbiology Reviews* 16, no. 3 (July 2003): 463–96.

26. Tyler Wheeler, "What Is a Pseudomonas Infection?" MedicineNet website, accessed January 21, 2022.

27. Shmuel Shoham, "Aspergillus," Poc-It Guides, Johns Hopkins Medicine website, accessed January 21, 2022.

28. Rebecca A. Drummond, "Candida albicans," British Society for Immunology website, accessed January 21, 2022.

29. "HIV/AIDS," Mayo Clinic website, accessed January 21, 2022.

CHAPTER 6. HABITS THAT HURT,
HABITS THAT HELP

1. Firdhaus S. Dabhar, "Effects of Stress on Immune System Function: The Good, the Bad, and the Beautiful," *Immunologic Research* 58, no. 2–3 (May 2014): 193–210.

2. G. Pawelec, A. Akbar, C. Caruso, R. Solana, B. Grubeck-Loebenstein, and A. Wikby, "Human Immunosenescence: Is It Infectious?" *Immunological Reviews* 205 (2005): 257–68.

3. Jennifer N. Morey et al., "Current Directions in Stress and Human Immune Function," *Current Opinions in Psychology* 5 (October 1, 2015): 13–17.

4. Danny J. J. Wang et al., "Cerebral Blood Flow Changes Associated with Different Meditation Practices and Perceived Depth of Meditation," *Psychiatry Research* 191, no. 1 (January 30, 2011): 60–67.

5. Ramy Abou Ghayda et al., "Correlations of Clinical and Laboratory Characteristics of COVID-19: A Systematic Review and Meta-Analysis," *International Journal of Environmental Research and Public Health* 17, no. 14 (July 13, 2020): 5026.

6. Michael R. Irwin, "Why Sleep Is Important for Health: A Psychoneuroimmunology Perspective," *Annual Review of Psychology* 66 (January 3, 2015): 143–72.

Index